AF333480

Extracorporeal Renal Surgery and Autotransplantation

Springer
Berlin
Heidelberg
New York
Barcelona
Budapest
Hong Kong
London
Milan
Paris
Santa Clara
Singapore
Tokyo

Inge B. Brekke
Audun Flatmark (Eds.)

Extracorporeal Renal Surgery and Autotransplantation

With Contributions by

D. Albrechtsen · Ø. H. Bentdal · H. Bondevik · I. B. Brekke
P. Fauchald · J. G. Fjeld · A. Flatmark · A. Foss
A. Hartmann · H. Holdaas · R. Innes · A. Jakobsen
N. E. Kløw · B. Lien · O. Øyen · P. F. Pfeffer · K. Rootwelt
G. Sødal and K. Vatne

With 51 Figures (in 99 Separate Illustrations) and 20 Tables

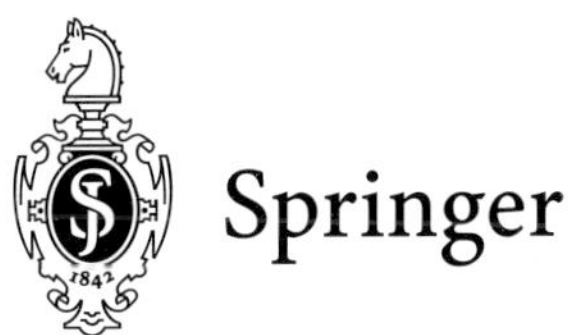

Springer

Inge B. Brekke, MD, PhD
Head of Transplant Surgery
Transplant Section, Department of Surgery
Rikshospitalet (The National Hospital)
University of Oslo, Pilestredet 32
N-0027 Oslo, Norway

Audun Flatmark, MD, PhD
Professor Emeritus
Department of Surgery
Rikshospitalet (The National Hospital)
University of Oslo, Pilestredet 32
N-0027 Oslo, Norway

ISBN 3-540-62761-8 Springer-Verlag Berlin Heidelberg New York

Library of Congress Cataloging-in-Publication Data. Extracorporeal renal surgery and autotransplantation / Inge B. Brekke, Audun Flatmark (eds.) ; with contributions by D. Albrechtsen . . . [et al.] p. cm. Includes bibliographical references and index. ISBN 3-540-62761-8 (Hardcover : alk. paper) 1. Kidney – Surgery. 2. Kidneys – Transplantation. 3. Autotransplantation. I. Brekke, Inge B., 1938– . II. Flatmark, Audrun, 1921– . III. Albrechtsen, Dagfinn. [DNML: 1. Kidney – surgery. 2. Kidney Transplantation – methods. 3. Transplantation, Autologous – methods. WJ 368 E96 1997] RD575.E95 1997 617.5'562–dc21 DNLM/DLC for Library of Congress 97-17144 CIP

Cover design: Erich Kirchner, Heidelberg

Typesetting: Verlagsservice Teichmann, 69256 Mauer

SPIN: 10502915   21/3155/SPS – 5 4 3 2 1 0 – Printed on acid-free paper

Preface

Some transplant centers have adopted bench surgery and subsequent renal autotransplantation as a regular policy in the treatment of a variety of renal disorders. The center in Gothenburg was among the first to start using this technique. My close friend, the late Lars-Erik (Charlie) Gelin, who headed the Gothenburg clinic until 1980, was enthusiastic about the method. We had many discussions and exchanged results. The method has proven to be safe and has saved many patients from becoming uremic. We have both been strong advocates of the use of this technique.

I performed my first renal autograft in April 1973. A 28-year-old man presented with hypertension (270/180 mm Hg), foggy vision, and a serum creatinine concentration of 400 mmol/l. The main artery to the right kidney was occluded, but an accessory artery to the lower pole was open. The left kidney was nonfunctioning and, weighing only 20 g, it was later removed. The right kidney was taken to a side table. The thrombus in the right renal artery was removed and the kidney was flushed and retransplanted. The patient is now 53 years of age with a blood pressure of 125/90 and a serum creatinine concentration of 137 µmol/l. Extracorporeal renal surgery with subsequent autotransplantation saved him from uremia and the need for a kidney allotransplant and has subsequently saved many another patient.

By the end of November 1996, we had autografted more than 500 kidneys in 479 patients. In spite of shock wave techniques and endoscopy in the treatment of stone disease and PTRA for renovascular disease, we still regularly receive patients for bench surgery, particularly patients with renal or urothelial carcinoma.

The present book summarizes our experience through the end of 1995. Inge B. Brekke, the present head of the transplant program, had the idea of writing this book 2 years ago. He has been the coordinator in the process, and I personally owe him many thanks.

The editors acknowledge the cooperation of all contributors to this book. We are indebted to Ms Siv K. Nielsen for her excellent secretarial assistance and to Ms Kari Toverud for her fine and skillfully performed anatomical illustrations. We also thank The Norwegian Medical Association Funds for Quality Improvement and Medinnova, Rikshospitalet, for their financial support. The patience demonstrated by the Springer-Verlag staff during the processing of this book has been highly appreciated.

AUDUN FLATMARK
December 1996

Table of Contents

1 **Effects of Renovascular Disease and Autotransplantation on Blood Pressure and Renal Function**
Anders Hartmann, Per Fauchald, and Hallvard Holdaas

1.1 Renovascular Disease 1
1.1.1 Renovascular Hypertension 1
1.1.2 Renal Dysfunction Associated with Renovascular Disease 4
1.2 Effects of Renal Autotransplantation on Overall Renal Function 8
1.2.1 General Considerations 8
1.2.2 Denervation and Reinnervation 9
1.2.3 Adaptive Changes in the Autotransplanted Kidney 15
References

2 **Radiological Investigation and Interventional Procedures in Patients with Renal Artery Disease**
Nils Einar Kløw and Karleif Vatne 21

2.1 Introduction 21
2.2 Screening Methods 21
2.3 Preoperative Investigation 22
2.3.1 Arteriography 22
2.3.2 Intravenous Digital Subtraction Angiography 25
2.3.3 Magnetic Resonance Angiography 25
2.3.4 Computed Tomographic Angiography 25
2.3.5 Duplex Doppler Imaging 26
2.4 Postoperative Investigations 27
2.5 Percutaneous Transluminal Renal Angioplasty 30
2.5.1 Percutaneous Transluminal Renal Angioplasty of the In Situ Kidney 31
2.5.2 Percutaneous Transluminal Renal Angioplasty of the Autotransplanted Kidney 32
2.6 Conclusions 35
References 35

3 **Renal Radionuclide Studies**
Jan G. Fjeld and Kjell Rootwelt 37

3.1 Introduction 37
3.1.1 Radiopharmaceuticals 37
3.1.2 Equipment 38

3.2   Basic Principles for Quantitative Evaluation 39
3.2.1   Blood Sampling Methods 39
3.2.2   Extrarenal Surface Activity Measurement 39
3.2.3   Kidney Uptake 39
3.2.4   Transit Times 40
3.3   Clinical Procedures: Methodology 41
3.3.1   Glomerular Filtration Rate 41
3.3.2   Renography 41
3.3.3   Intervention Renographies 42
3.3.4   Autotransplant Renography 43
3.4   Selected Procedures in Preoperative Work-up 43
3.4.1   Renovascular Disease 43
3.4.2   Urinary Obstruction 45
3.4.3   Renal Cancer 45
3.5   Autotransplant Follow-up 45
3.5.1   Total Renal Function 45
3.5.2   Autotransplant Function 49
         References 49

4   **Nephrectomy and Extracorporeal Renal Preservation: Technical Details**
         Bjørn Lien and Inge B. Brekke 51

4.1   Preoperative Evaluation and Preparation 51
4.2   Anatomical Considerations 51
4.3   Nephrectomy: Technical Details 53
4.3.1   Choice of Incision 53
4.3.2   Nephrectomy for Nonmalignant Disease 56
4.3.3   Nephrectomy for Renal Carcinoma 57
4.4   Extracorporeal Renal Preservation 59
         References

5   **Renal Autotransplantation: Indications, Basic Surgical Techniques,**
         and Complications
         Inge B. Brekke and Gunnar Sødal 63

5.1   Introduction and Historical Background 63
5.2   Indications 64
5.3   Basic Surgical Techniques 64
5.3.1   Extracorporeal Preparation of the Kidney 64
5.3.2   Kidney Replantation 66
5.4.   Complications 71
5.4.1   Vascular Complications 72
5.4.2   Urological Complications 72
         References 72

6   **Renal Artery Atherosclerosis**
Aksel Foss, Arnt Jakobsen, and Dagfinn Albrechtsen 77

6.1   Introduction 77
6.2   Atherosclerotic Renal Artery Disease: The Natural Story 79
6.3   Management of Blood Pressure in Atherosclerotic RVH 79
6.4   Percutaneous Transluminal Renal Angioplasty vs Surgery 80
6.5   Surgical Management of Atherosclerotic Renal Artery Disease 81
6.6   Renal Autotransplantation in Atherosclerotic Renal Disease 83
6.7   Summary 84
          References

7   **The Role of Bench Surgery in the Treatment of Renal**
Artery Stenoses and Aneurysms Caused by Fibromuscular Dysplasia
Inge B. Brekke and Bjørn Lien 87

7.1   Introduction 87
7.2   Diagnosis 89
7.3   Indications for Surgery 90
7.3.1   Hypertension 90
7.3.2   Preservation and Restoration of Renal Function 91
7.3.3   Loin Pain/Hematuria Syndrome 92
7.4   Choice of Surgical Technique 92
7.5   Extracorporeal Renal Artery Reconstruction 93
7.6   Renal Reimplantation and Postoperative Control 95
7.7   Results 95
7.7.1   Effect on Hypertension 95
7.7.2   Effect on Kidney Function 96
7.7.3   Surgical Complications 96
7.7.4   Patient Survival 97
7.8   Conclusion 97
          References 98

8   **Complicated Renal Calculous Disease Treated by Extracorporeal Surgery**
and Autotransplantation
Per F. Pfeffer, Helge Bondevik, and Gunnar Sødal 101

8.1   Introduction 101
8.2   Indications for Extracorporeal Surgery 101
8.3   Preoperative Examination and Evaluation 103
8.4   Surgical Procedures 104
8.5   Postoperative Follow up 107
8.6   Results 108
8.6.1   Recurrence of Calculi 109
8.6.2   Autotransplant Function 109
8.6.3   Postoperative Complications 110
8.7   Summary 111
          References 111

9   Ex Vivo Renal Resection and Autotransplantation for Renal and Urothelial Carcinoma
Gunnar Sødal, Øystein Bentdal, and Audun Flatmark 113

9.1   Introduction 113
9.2   Indications for Extracorporeal Surgery 113
9.3   Surgical Technique 113
9.3.1   Preparation of the Kidney (Bench Surgery) 114
9.4   Postoperative Follow-Up 119
9.5   Own Experience 119
9.6   Results 120
9.6.1   Perioperative Complications 120
9.6.2   Long-Term Results 121
9.7   Discussion 122
         References

10   Simultaneous Aortic Reconstruction and Renal Autotransplantation
Inge B. Brekke, Ole Øyen, Robert Innes, and Audun Flatmark 125

10.1   Introduction 125
10.2   Prevalence of Aortorenal Disease 126
10.2.1   Juxta- and Pararenal Aortic Aneurysms 126
10.2.2   Coexistent Aortic and Renal Artery Disease 127
10.3   Indications for a Combined Procedure 128
10.4   Preoperative Assessment 128
10.5   Surgery 129
10.5.1   Peroperative Management 129
10.5.2   Aortic Replacement and Renal Autotransplantation 130
10.6   Postoperative Care and Evaluation 131
10.7   Results 133
10.7.1   Perioperative Morbidity and Mortality 133
10.7.2   Effect on Blood Pressure and Renal Function 133
10.8   Summary 134
         References 135

11   Management of Ureteral Defects by Renal Autotransplantation
Øystein H. Bentdal and Gunnar Sødal 139

11.1   Introduction 139
11.2   Alternative Surgical Techniques 139
11.3   Own Experience 139
11.4   Results 140
11.5   Summary 142
         References 142

Subject Index 143

Contributors

All authors, except Helge Bondevik, are staff of Rikshospitalet (The National Hospital), University of Oslo, Pilestredet 32, 0027 Oslo, Norway.

Albrechtsen, Dagfinn, MD, PhD
Consultant Transplant Surgeon and Assistant Medical Director
Transplant Section, Department of Surgery

Bentdal, Øystein H., MD, PhD
Consultant Transplant Surgeon
Transplant Section, Department of Surgery

Bondevik, Helge, MD, PhD
Consultant Transplant Surgeon
Now Consultant Vascular Surgeon
Bærum County Hospital, Bærum

Brekke, Inge B., MD, PhD
Head of Transplant Surgery
Transplant Section, Department of Surgery

Fauchald, Per, MD, PhD
Professor of Nephrology
Head of Nephrology Section
Department of Medicine

Fjeld, Jan G., MD, M.Sc., PhD
Consultant
Section for Nuclear Medicine
Department of Clinical Chemistry

Flatmark Audun, MD, PhD
Professor Emeritus
Department of Surgery

Foss, Aksel, MD, PhD
Consultant Transplant Surgeon
Transplant Section, Department of Surgery

Hartmann, Anders, MD, PhD
Consultant
Nephrology Section, Department of Medicine

Holdaas, Hallvard, MD, PhD
Consultant
Nephrology Section, Department of Medicine

Innes, Robert, MD
Consultant
Department of Anesthesiology

Jakobsen, Arnt, M.D., PhD
Consultant transplant surgeon,
Department of Surgery
Present position Medical Director

Kløw, Nils Einar, MD, PhD
Consultant
Department of Radiology
Present address:
Department of Radiology
University of Minnesota
Box 292 UMHC, 420 Delaware Street S.E., MN 55455, USA

Lien, Bjørn, MD
Consultant Transplant Surgeon
Transplant Section, Department of Surgery

Øyen, Ole, MD, PhD
Consultant Transplant Surgeon
Transplant Section, Department of Surgery

Pfeffer, Per F., MD, PhD
Consultant Transplant Surgeon
Transplant Section, Department of Surgery

Rootwelt, Kjell, MD, PhD
Professor of Nuclear Medicine
Head of Section for Nuclear Medicine
Department of Clinical Chemistry

Sødal, Gunnar, MD
Consultant Transplant Surgeon
Transplant Section, Department of Surgery

Vatne, Karleif, MD
Consultant
Department of Radiology

Effects of Renovascular Disease and Autotransplantation on Blood Pressure and Renal Function

Anders Hartmann, Per Fauchald, and Hallvard Holdaas

1.1
Renovascular Disease

1.1.1
Renovascular Hypertension

1.1.1.1
Prevalence and Diagnosis

Renovascular hypertension (RVH) is estimated to be prevalent in ca. 0.5%-1% of the total hypertensive population. The percentage recorded depends on the diagnostic criteria used and the selection of patients screened. Reported prevalence of RVH is 2%-4% in patients referred to hospitals or other specialist investigation, increasing to 5%-15% in therapy-resistant hypertension and up to 35% in accelerated or malignant hypertension (Lüscher and Kaplan 1992).

The diagnosis cannot solely be based on the demonstration of a vascular stenosis as a substantial proportion of elderly normotensives (45% over the age of 60 years) have angiographic evidence of renal vascular disease. Postmortem examination has even shown a prevalence of 70% (Eyler et al. 1962; Holley et al. 1964). Improvement or cure of hypertension after relief of renal vascular obstruction is of course the ultimate proof of RVH.

1.1.1.2
Screening Procedures

Several noninvasive techniques have been introduced to screen for RVH and to evaluate the physiological significance of an anatomical lesion in the renal artery. These functional investigations are based on activation of the renin-angiotensin system, either by measuring the hormone levels in renal venous blood in peripheral circulation or by measuring changes in the glomerular filtration rate or renal blood flow.

From the middle of the 1980s several clinical studies (Sfakianakis et al. 1987; Pedersen 1994) have suggested that angiotensin coverting enzyme inhibitor (ACE inhibitor) renography may be used to diagnose RVH with a positive and negative predictive diagnostic value ranging between 80% and 90%. Aspirin renography, another of the newer approaches for screening renovascular hypertension, also appears promising (Bubeck 1995). Conventional renography without ACE inhibitor has a lower positive predictive value, while the ratio of renin activity in the renal veins has a lower negative predictive value.

Based on clinical criteria (severe and refractory hypertension, onset of hypertension before the age of 25 years and after the age of 45 years, abrupt progression of hypertension, abdominal or flank bruit, peripheral vascular disease and abnormal serum creatinine) it is possible to select patients with a high (22%-51%) likelihood of RVH (Svetkey et al. 1991; Setaro et al. 1991). These selected patients should be screened for RVH. Currently it seems that ACE inhibitor renography is the preferred method. In some patients with a high clinical suspicion of RVH, angiographic examination could be performed without other primary screening. As the angiographic finding of renal artery obstruction is a sine qua non for the diagnosis of RVH, it could be discussed whether angiography as the primary diagnostic procedure in selected patients is more cost-effective than using one of the less invasive screening methods.

It is difficult to evaluate the value of functional screening methods in predicting whether active treatment with either percutaneous transluminal renal angioplasty (PTRA) or surgery results in cure or improvement of blood pressure regulation. The available studies are relatively modest in size and definitions of cure or improvement differ. It seems, however, that an abnormal ACE inhibitor renogram in a patient with RVH is a good predictor of successful revascularization results and that a negative ACE inhibitor renogram before PTRA predicts poor results (Pedersen 1994).

1.1.1.3
Conservative Treatment vs Intervention

When RVH is diagnosed anatomically and functionally (by ACE inhibitor renography or by some other screening method) a choice between medical treatment or a revascularization procedure must be made. The indication for preserving or improving renal function in patients with bilateral renal artery obstruction or renal artery stenosis in a solitary kidney is discussed below. In unilateral RVH with a normal contralateral kidney, medical management will usually adequately control blood pressure in the majority of patients (see Table 1.1), but the underlying obstructive process may progress and the patient has to continue a life-long antihypertensive medication. The major factors to consider in such patients when selecting treatment modalities, include the etiology of the stenosis (fibrous/fibromuscular vs atherosclerotic), associated cardiovascular and cerebrovascular disease, age, adequacy of blood pressure control, side-effects of the medical treatment, and cost. Patients with fibromuscular disease tend to be young and, although the most common form (medial fibroplasia) rarely progresses to occlusion, these patients should primarily be considered for PTRA, and if unsuccessful, they are generally excellent candidates for surgical revascularization. In this context it should be remembered that all forms of fibrous disease can progress with involvement of the contralateral kidney. Atherosclerotic renal artery stenosis represents a more complex situation. The patients are usually elderly with associated vascular disease. The rate of renal artery occlusion has been reported as high as 40% (Sos 1991). In other studies the occlusion rate is much lower, ranging from 12% to 16%, (Dean et al 1968; Schreiber et al. 1984). However, all studies are small and the follow-up times differ. It is, however, well documented that there is a substantial risk of occlusion and of progression of changes in the contralateral kidney. PTRA is the treatment of choice in unilateral nonostial renal lesion, leaving a low complication rate and a high anatomical success rate. In ostial lesions PTRA should be considered as the primary treatment, if necessary, supplemented by stent insertion. If not applicable or unsuccessful, surgical intervention may be considered. Because of the inferior results of PTRA in ostial lesions, the indications should be restricted to high risk patients (extensive atherosclerotic disease, high age).

In most cases surgical revascularization is reserved for patients unsuccessfully treated by PTRA supplemented by stent when indicated. All candidates for surgery should be screened for coronary heart disease by exercise ECG and/or stress thallium scans. Doppler examination of the carotid arteries and, if coronary heart disease is suspected, coronary angiography should be performed. High-risk patients should receive medical treatment. It is currently held that increased glomerular efferent arteriolar tone, maintained by angiotensin II (AII), supports the glomerular filtration rate (GFR) in kidneys with reduced perfusion pressure caused by renal artery stenosis. Deterioration in GFR has been associated with ACE inhibitor treatment. In some cases with bilateral renal artery stenosis or stenosis of the artery to a single functioning kidney reversible anuria and even occlusion has been described. However, ACE inhibitors are effective in RVH, and in unilateral renal artery stenosis they may be used with caution as initial therapy. Calcium channel blockers are also effective and safe in RVH. As a third option, beta blockers or diuretics may be used as required (Rosenthal 1993). If multiple antihypertensive drugs are needed, if blood pressure control is poor or the function in the affected kidney is declining, the patient should be reevaluated for PTRA or surgical intervention. The treatment options are summarized in Table 1.1.

Table 1.1. Treatment options for consideration

	Relative effects	
	Cholesterol	Triglycerides

I. Medical
  Antihypertensive treatment
    ACE-inhibitors
    Calcium channel inhibitors
    Beta- or Alpha-/betablockers
    Combination/others
  Lipid-lowering drugs
    HMG-CoA reductase inhibitors (statins) — Cholesterol +++, Triglycerides +
    Bile-acid sequestrants — Cholesterol ++, Triglycerides –
    Nicotinic acid — Cholesterol ++, Triglycerides ++
    Probucol — Cholesterol ++
    Fibric acid derivatives — Cholesterol +, Triglycerides +++
    Omega 3-fatty acids — Cholesterol –, Triglycerides +(+)
  Anticoagulant therapy
    Aspirin (ASA)
    Other "anti-platelet" drugs
    Coumarin derivates

II. Life-style changes (prophylactic)
  Cessation of smoking
  Diet (lipid-lowering)
  Physical activity

III. Direct vascular intervention options
  Percutaneous transluminal renal angioplasty (PTRA)
    Intraarterial stenting if necessary
  Surgical vascular reconstruction/autotransplantation

1.1.2
Renal Dysfunction Associated with Renovascular Disease

1.1.2.1
Pathogenesis

Renovascular disease as a cause of hypertension, its diagnosis and its effect of treatment as discussed above, have been thoroughly investigated for 60 years since the first experimental study on experimental renovascular hypertension was published by Goldblatt et al. (1934). However, the impact of obstructive vascular disease on renal function itself has only recently gained attention (Scoble and Hamilton 1990; Pohl 1993). Although glomerular filtration is autoregulated and may be sustained during substantial reduction in renal perfusion pressure, widespread atherosclerosis of the vasculature may also include the autoregulatory segments, implicating the arcuate arteries, interlobular arteries, and arterioles (Heyeraas and Aukland 1987). In any case a major obstruction of the upstream vasculature may reduce glomerular perfusion pressure below the autoregulatory range with ensuing glomerular hypofiltration.

In a clinical situation dysfunction in one of two functioning kidneys may well be neglected as the serum creatinine often remains within the normal range and may be so even if one kidney is severely affected or nonfunctioning. This is consistent with the finding that there is usually a normal serum creatinine following donor nephrectomy (Talseth et al. 1986; Najarian et al. 1992). On the other hand, with bilateral renal vascular disease, a clinically significant reduction in kidney function is more likely to appear. Atherosclerosis is often a generalized disease, especially in the elderly. Forty per cent of patients over 50 years of age suffering from single atherosclerotic artery stenosis develop contralateral disease in the course of 4 years (Scoble and Hamilton 1990).

It is conceivable that the reduction in kidney function starts as a reversible process due to the reduction in glomerular perfusion pressure. Obviously, with arterial occlusion or long-term severe ischemia, glomerulosclerosis and interstitial scarring ensues, with a permanent reduction in kidney function.

1.1.2.2
Diagnosis and Nomenclature

The International Classification of Diseases (ICD9) does not carry a diagnosis of "ischemic kidney disease," probably because of the relatively new concept of renal ischemic dysfunction However, the most recent ICD10 version soon to be implemented, contains a diagnosis "N28.0 - ischemia and infarction of the kidney" that may adequately address the phenomenon of renal dysfunction caused by renovascular renal disease, even when hypertension is modest or nonexistent. The diagnosis of renovascular disease in the absence of hypertension is usually established randomly during invasive angiography for investigation of other diseases. In some cases clinical suspicion may be aroused by a rise in serum creatinine in a patient with generalized atherosclerotic disease.

1.1.2.2.1
Random Diagnosis by Angiography

Renal artery disease has traditionally been suspected and diagnosed as a cause of secondary hypertension. The widespread and increasing use of diagnostic angiography in suspected coronary heart disease has uncovered a large group of patients with renovascular disease without renovascular hypertension. In most cases the kidney function appears normal. If the vasculature of both kidneys is affected, serum creatinine may be elevated (Sos 1991; Martin et al. 1987; Scoble and Hamilton 1990; Dean et al. 1991).

1.1.2.2.2
Diagnosis Through Declining Renal Function

Most nephrologists do not primarily address renal vascular disease as a primary cause of progressive decline in renal function unless there is prevailing hypertension. A renal angiogram is only likely to be performed if a kidney biopsy reveals ischemic changes and/or infarctions. However, a more systematic search for underlying renal vascular disease may be warranted, especially if no other specific diagnosis is established. In a population of more than 100 patients over 50 years of age presenting with advanced renal failure , the underlying cause was renal vascular disease in 14% of the cases (Scoble and Hamilton 1990).

1.1.2.3
Long-Term Consequences of Obstructed Blood Flow for Renal Function

What are the consequences of long-term renal vascular impairment in the absence of renovascular hypertension? This is a crucial question when considering intervention. Data are scarce on renal survival in normotensive patients with renovascular disease. The most serious consequence is obviously renal artery occlusion leading to infarction of the kidney. However, because of extrarenal collateral blood supply, the kidney, although practically nonfiltering, may survive and remain in a "hibernating state." Kidney function has been rescued in some cases even when revascularization was performed after several months (Pohl 1993; Schefft et al. 1980; Novick 1991). This may be regarded as a parallel to the state of cardial "hibernation" following coronary artery obstruction or occlusion with the notable exception that the kidneys are paired organs. With one remaining kidney the overall renal function may still be adequate. However, atherosclerosis often prevails in the vasculature of the remaining kidney, leaving the patient at high risk for future development of renal end-stage disease (Scoble and Hamilton 1990).

It has been shown that a diameter stenosis of 50% (75% area) of a major artery implies significant hypoperfusion, but thrombosis of the artery may occur also with smaller atherosclerotic lesions (Textor 1994). Knowledge of the incidence of spontaneous development of renal vascular occlusion is limited. A review of three different studies reveal a 13%-40% chance for occlusion of a significantly stenosed renal artery over as little as 1 year (Sos 1991). There is a lack of data on the rate of progression of renal failure caused by more generalized renal vascular atherosclerotic disease distal to the main renal artery. We believe that the importance of renovascular disease as a cause of progressive loss of kidney function in general is underestimated.

1.1.2.4
Therapy

Therapeutic options include conservative measures versus direct vascular intervention/reconstruction. The different choices of therapy summarized below are (except for antihypertensive drugs) the same as for renovascular hypertension (see Table 1.1).

1.1.2.4.1
Conservative Treatment

The effects of the noninvasive measures involving lifestyle and medical intervention have not been adequately evaluated for renal atherosclerosis and its complications. We find it reasonable, however, to apply conservative measures in this patient group as accepted for patients with generalized atherosclerosis and reviewed elsewhere (Pyörälä et al. 1994). Such measures are applied differently throughout the world. Since the majority of these patients also suffer from generalized atherosclerotic and coronary heart disease, conservative treatment should imply anticoagulant therapy (usually acetylsalicylic acid; ASA) and lipid-lowering drugs at relatively modest elevations of total cholesterol or low-density lipoprotein cholesterol (LDL cholesterol); such treatment has recently been shown to reduce mortality by 30% in patients with symptomatic coronary heart disease (The Scandinavian simvastatin survival study group 1994).

1.1.2.4.2
Direct Vascular Intervention

The long-term effect on renal function of revascularization either by angioplasty or surgery has not been elucidated in prospective randomized trials. However, since as many as 40% of patients with significant renal arterial stenosis may experience arterial occlusion within a year (Sos 1991), it is conceivable that a successful revascularization procedure in many of these patients would be a "kidney saving" procedure. The effect of renal arterial angioplasty on renal functional preservation has been addressed in several retrospective studies (Sos 1991; Martin et al. 1987; Bell et al. 1987; Pattynama et al. 1994). Figure 1.1, adapted from Martin et al. (1987), shows the success rates with regard to improvement of renal function at different levels of azotemia. Improvement of renal function was defined as a fall in serum creatinine of more than 20%. The overall success rate in the different studies varies from 30% to 47% and was even higher if only patients with technically successful angioplasty procedures were evaluated (Sos 1991). It is important to note that the success rates were considerably lower when renal function was substantially reduced, especially with a serum creatinine higher than 400 mmol/l. The positive effect on kidney function could be demonstrated up to 1-3 years following the procedure (Martin et al. 1987; Bell et al. 1987; Sos 1991; Pattynama et al. 1994). The nephrotoxic effect of the radiographic contrast agent itself

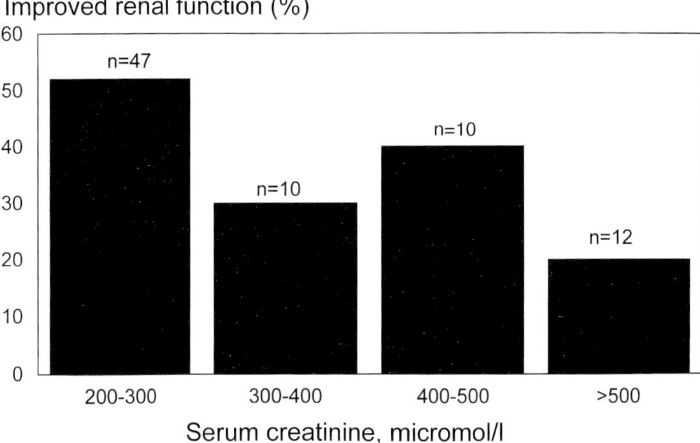

Fig. 1.1. Percentage of patients with improved renal function following percutaneous transluminal renal angioplasty (PTRA). The patient groups are stratified according to serum creatinine levels prior to PTRA. (Adapted from Martin et al. 1987, with permission)

may partly explain the lack of positive effect in patients with severely compromised kidney function (Harkonen and Kjellstrand 1981). Angioplasty was performed on both single and bilateral renal artery stenosis as well as in cases with stenosis of a single functioning kidney. The best results were obtained in patients with bilateral renal vascular stenosis. Most of the patients studied had some degree of hypertension. Studies on selected normotensive patients with significant renovascular disease have not been performed. Some degree of hypertension is often present and diagnostic tests for renovascular hypertension may be inconclusive. However, an ongoing prospective study addresses the effect of revascularization on the preservation of renal function (Pohl 1993). Patients with significant renal arterial stenoses without renovascular hypertension are randomized to either conservative treatment or to direct vascular intervention. No differences had been observed between the groups by the end of 1991 (43 patients).

In recent years, the policy at our center has been to encourage angioplasty in cases of significant lesions suitable for angioplasty in one or several renal arteries. Lesions on branches of one or several renal arteries have only rarely been treated with angioplasty and renovascular surgery and autotransplantation has only been applied in a few highly selected patients in order to preserve renal function. The results of renal vascular angioplasty in more than 400 patients at our center are now under validation. Only a few of these were performed primarily in an effort to sustain or improve kidney function. Furthermore our large series points towards a high percentage of salvage of renal function except at high serum creatinine levels (Paulsen et al. 1996).

The role of surgical intervention in renovascular atherosclerotic lesions is discussed in a separate chapter of this book. It is notable that renovascular surgery for preservation of kidney function has been encouraging even with ostial and multiple peripheral arterial lesions unsuited to angioplasty (Pohl et al. 1991; Sos 1991; Dean et al. 1991; Novick 1991; Textor 1994).

1.2
Effects of Renal Autotransplantation on Overall Renal Function

1.2.1
General Considerations

Autotransplantation and extracorporeal surgery of the kidney implies resection of the vascular stalk containing not only the renal artery and vein but also the lymphatic network draining the kidney, as well as afferent and efferent renal nerves. The effect of denervation on different aspects of renal function will be dealt with below. The impact on lymphatic outflow from the kidney does not normally affect kidney function or blood pressure. However, because of the excised lymph vessels, renal allotransplantation is complicated in some 10% of cases by the development of a lymphocele that may compress and obstruct the urine flow and thus impair renal function. By contrast, a lymphocele does not as a rule develop following renal autotransplantation as discussed elsewhere in this book (see Chap. 5).

1.2.1.1
One vs Two Functioning Kidneys

Obviously the effect of renal autotransplantation on overall kidney function depends on whether one or both kidneys are autotransplanted. Of course, a solitary functioning kidney may also be autotransplanted. The most common situation is autotransplantation of one kidney with a normally functioning contralateral kidney. The reason may be a unilateral renal arterial lesion or a renal carcinoma. If technically successful the impact on the function of the kidneys, blood pressure, and salt and water homeostasis is probably negligible. However, in patients with a single functioning kidney or with a remaining severely dysfunctioning kidney, functional changes may be seen. The effects of renal autotransplantation and allotransplantation on kidney function are the same in principle.

The lesson learnt from renal allografting is that the overall impact of the transplantation per se is small when it comes to blood pressure regulation and salt and fluid balance. Blood pressure elevation in allotransplanted patients is usually related to the use of cyclosporine or preexisting hypertension (Kasiske 1987). Nevertheless the effects of the autotransplantation procedure itself on renal function is of considerable theoretical interest and may be of importance under certain circumstances, as will be discussed below.

1.2.1.2
The Role of Renal Function

Obviously the prospects for maintaining renal function depend on the degree of renal parenchymal injury. Consistent with what has previously been discussed, the renal vascular disease may render the kidney ischemic, but alive in a "hibernating" state. In such cases the chances for salvage of renal function are outstanding (Sos 1991; Dean et al. 1991; Martin et al. 1987; Pickering 1991).

If the parenchyma suffers permanent damage due to infarctions and sclerosis, only partial improvement at best may be expected. The same would be the case with concurrent kidney disease unrelated to renovascular disease. Finally, resection of kidney tissue due to carcinoma or calcification, as discussed in a separate chapter, obviously impairs the functional outcome. However, adequate renal function may be obtained even following extensive surgical excisions of the kidney (Novick et al. 1991).

1.2.1.3
Ischemia Time

Organ preservation methods have been developed for allotransplantation, allowing successful cadaveric kidney transplantation exposed to cold ischemia for more than 30 h. The cold ischemia time associated with extracorporeal bench surgery of the kidney is usually less than 2 h (Novick 1991). Consequently the limited ischemia time during proper extracorporeal surgery and autotransplantation probably has little or no effect on long-term renal function.

1.2.2
Denervation and Reinnervation

There is an extensive adrenergic innervation of the kidney which provides a regulatory mechanism for acute and chronic response of the kidney to homeostatic requirements. The renal nerves play an important role in modulating systemic blood pressure; they regulate renal vascular resistance and thereby renal blood flow and glomerular filtration rate, modulate tubular solute and water transport, and influence secretion of renin (Kopp et al. 1984). These aspects are dealt with in more detail below.

1.2.2.1
Renal Neuroanatomy

Electron microscope and histochemical fluorescence methods have demonstrated a rich sympathetic innervation of the kidney (Barajas et al. 1992). Renal efferent nerves extend from the celiac plexus, the thoracic and lumbar branches of the splanchnic nerves, the superior and inferior mesenteric plexus, the intermesenteric nerves, and the superior hypogastric plexus (Mitchell 1950). These nerve fibers constitute the renal plexus from which nerves follow the renal vessels to enter the hilus of the kidney. Efferent renal nerves form a network around the afferent and efferent arterioles, the renin-secreting juxtaglomerular cells and the cortical tubules (Barajas 1978). The tubular innervation include the proximal tubules, the thick ascending limb of Henle, the distal convoluted tubules, and the collecting ducts (Barajas et al. 1984). Innervation is most dense in the ascending limb of Henle, followed by the distal convoluted tubule and the proximal tubule. Norepinephrine is the transmitter at the terminal of the postganglionic peripheral nerves, although dopamine is present within all noradrenergic axons as a transmitter precursor (Kopp and DiBona 1992). However, functional studies of the dog kidney do not support the existence of functionally significant renal dopaminergic innervation (Holdaas and DiBona 1984).

Afferent impulses from the kidney are mediated via myelinated and unmyelinated fibers, the unmyelinated fibers having a predominant role in afferent renal innervation (Knuepfer and Schramm 1987). The afferent renal nerves arise from intrarenal sensory receptors and project to the central nervous system. Two types of receptors exist, mechanoreceptors and chemoreceptors (Moss 1989). Several pharmacological agents have been found to stimulate the afferent nerves (Ferguson and Bell 1988; Miller et al. 1978).

1.2.2.2
Neural Control of Renal Function

1.2.2.2.1
Control of Renal Hemodynamics

Renal sympathetic nerve activity is important for physiological regulation of renal hemodynamics, tubular sodium and water reabsorption, and renin secretion. These effects constitute a control system in regulating arterial pressure as well as total body fluid and sodium homeostasis. The effects are summarized in Table 1.2.

Table 1.2. Renal sympathetic nerve activity

Renal nerve stimulation frequency (Hz)	Renal blood flow	Glomerular filtration rate	Renin Release	Sodium excretion
<0.25	o	o	Basal release: o Stimulated: ↑	o
0.25–1.0	o	o	↑	o
1.0–2.0	(↓)	o	↑↑	↓
>2.0	↓	↓	↑↑↑	↓

Basal renal nerve activity is generally too low to influence renal hemodynamics under normal physiologic conditions. Pharmacologic renal denervation in humans will normally not affect renal blood flow or glomerular filtration rate (Hollenberg et al. 1975). However, increased renal efferent sympathetic activity produces decreases in renal blood flow and glomerular filtration rate that are proportional to the magnitude of the increase in efferent sympathetic activity (Holdaas et al. 1981a). Thus the renal sympathetic nerves at basal conditions do not play a significant role in the autoregulation of renal blood flow, at least at modest physiological levels of renal sympathetic nerve activity. However, more intense degrees of renal sympathetic nerve stimulation or renal vascular a1-adrenoceptor stimulation are accompanied by an increase in the lowest autoregulatory pressure (Holdaas et al. 1981a; Langård et al. 1981). The a1-adrenoceptor is the predominating adrenoceptor subtype mediating renal vasoconstriction (Holdaas and DiBona 1984). The effects of renal sympathetic nerves on urinary sodium and water excretion are discussed below.

1.2.2.2.2
Control of Renin Release

There is considerable evidence that three primary mechanisms regulate renin release by the kidney; the renal vascular baroreceptor, the renal tubular macula densa receptor, and the renal sympathetic nerves (Kopp et al. 1984). The endogenous release of norepinephrine during efferent renal sympathetic nerve stimulation may increase renin release by activation of either a- or b-adrenoreceptors or both. Activation of a-adrenoreceptors of the renal vasculature results in renal vasoconstriction with reduced renal blood flow and glomerular filtration rate leading to a marked increase in renin release (Langaard et al. 1981). Low-frequency renal nerve stimulation (0.25 Hz), too low to produce any change in renal blood flow or glomerular filtration rate, is without effect on renin release at control blood pressure. However, by activation of the renal baroreceptors through reduction of the renal arterial pressure below the range of renal blood autoregulation or through the increase of ureteral pressure, low-frequency renal nerve stimulation increases renin release (Thames and DiBona 1979; Holdaas et al. 1981b). In the light of these observations it is clear that levels of efferent renal sympathetic nerve activity that do not affect renal hemodynamics or urinary sodium excretion can significantly augment the renin release response to nonneural stimuli, such as reductions in renal arterial pressure or increases in ureteral pressure. The clinical correlates of these experimental findings might be renal artery stenosis, systemic hypotension, and ureteral obstruction. Increasing evidence also suggests that renin release is modulated by low-pressure cardiac baroreceptor reflex with vagal afferent and renal efferent nerves. Unloading of cardiac baroreceptors with nonhypotensive hemorrhage results in an increase in renin secretion rate that is greater from the innervated than the contralateral denervated kidney and is abolished by renal denervation (Grandjean et al. 1978) or inflation of a balloon in the left atrium (Holdaas and DiBona 1981)

1.2.2.3
Functional Aspects of Renal Denervation

Renal denervation will not result in increased renal blood flow or glomerular filtration rate with normal basal renal nerve activity (Hollenberg et al. 1975; Sadowski et al. 1979). The capacity for autoregulation will also be unaffected by renal denervation. Basal renal sympathetic nerve activity thus has no influence on the resting tone of the renal vasculature.

Renal denervation will decrease basal and stimulated renin release. It is shown that renal denervation decreases messenger RNA for renin in experimental models (Zhang et al. 1992). These data indicate that a low basal level of renal sympathetic nerve activity has a tonic influence on basal renin synthesis and secretion. The basal level of activity of renal sympathetic nerves also has an influence on sodium and water excretion as discussed below.

1.2.2.4
Salt and Water Excretion

The acute effects of denervation provoking increased diuresis and salt excretion have long been recognized (Blake 1962). The direct and indirect effects of the renal nerves on renal sodium handling have been thoroughly investigated and reviewed elsewhere (Kopp and DiBona 1992). The denervation following renal transplantation may interfere with the homeostasis of salt and water via hemodynamic or tubular effects mediated either directly or indirectly via hormonal release. Renal hemodynamic effects from altered efferent sympathetic nerve traffic as discussed above may acutely affect the glomerular filtration rate and consequently the excretion of sodium (Kopp and DiBona 1992). Direct sympathetic innervation of different tubular segments has also been established (Barajas et al. 1984). Direct sodium conserving effects of efferent renal sympathetic nerves have been demonstrated in the dog, probably mediated via alpha-1 receptors in the proximal tubules (Osborn et al. 1983).

In the context of extracorporeal renal surgery and autotransplantation, it is important to note that these effects are relatively minor and with the other kidney intact probably negligible in a clinical situation. In the following only the effects of complete denervation of both kidneys or denervation of a single functioning kidney will be discussed.

1.2.2.4.1
Salt and Water Loading

Efferent renal nerve traffic promotes conservation of sodium and water in the kidney. Therefore autotransplantation of a kidney would not be expected to impair the capacity for excretion of loads of sodium and water. Experience from renal allografted patients has taught us that these patients are prone to suffer from ankle edema. They usually also show a tendency to water and salt overloading concomitant with low levels of plasma renin. Accordingly diuretics are commonly applied, especially in the early phase following transplantation. However, it is unlikely that these clinical findings are related to denervation of the graft. Except for a single early study in a single twin recipient and donor (Bricker et al. 1956), no evidence from renal allografting in man has demonstrated that renal denervation itself may provoke retention of salt and water (DiBona 1987). Salt and water retention in renal allografted patients is probably multifactorial. However, as illustrated in Fig. 1.2, experiments on conscious monkeys have shown that the acute excretion of sodium and water during the first few hours following a sodium reach meal was reduced by 30% after renal denervation (Peterson et al. 1991). It may therefore be concluded that the rapid excretion of salt and water following an acute salt load may be affected by denervation as has also been demonstrated in normotensive rats (Greenberg et al. 1991). The mechanism for such an effect has not been elucidated.

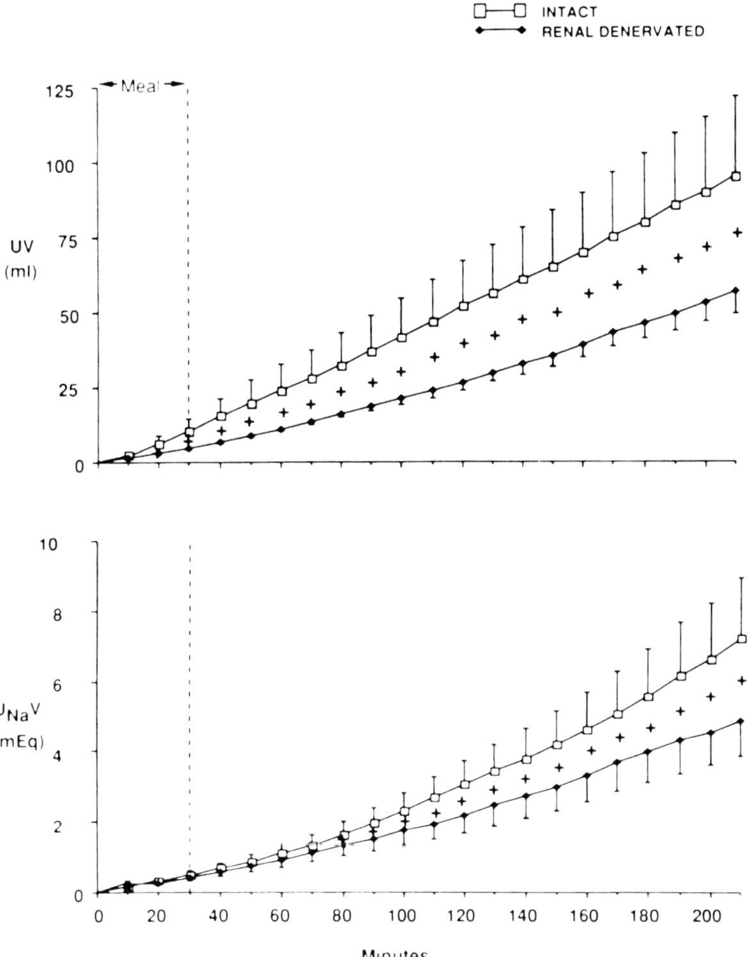

Fig. 1.2. Cumulative postprandial urine volume (UV) (upper panel) and the cumulative sodium excretion (UNaV) (lower panel) in conscious monkeys during the first hours following ingestion of a sodium-rich meal. Curves with open boxes denote intact animals. Black dotted curves show data from denervated animals. Significant difference between the groups is indicated by +. (From Peterson et al. 1991, with permission)

1.2.2.4.2
Salt Depletion

The major discussion related to denervation associated with renal transplantation has been focused on the ability of the kidney to preserve salt and volume during deprived intake.

Experimental studies in rats and dogs have yielded inconsistent results. A study in six living donor renal allografted recipients (Blaufox et al. 1969) demonstrated that the recipients were able to maintain sodium balance just as well as the donors during very low sodium intake (10 mmol daily). However, the recipients were examined up to several years following renal allografting and reinnervation might have occurred (DiBona 1987). By contrast patients suffering idiopathic or pharmacological autonomic nephropathy were not able to maintain sodium balance during sodium restriction (Gill and Barter 1966; Wilcox et al. 1977). It has therefore been concluded that renal nerve activity is functionally important during strict sodium retention (DiBona 1987). Experience from renal allografted patients has shown that clinical symptoms and signs of sodium depletion are relatively rare; on the contrary diuretics are usually given to avoid sodium and water retention during the first weeks and months. During chronic diuretic therapy a braking phenomenon is observed limiting diuretic effects over time. A relative resistance to the diuretic response develops, probably because of an intrinsic distal tubular adaptation during prolonged diuretic therapy. This may also involve hormonal and hemodynamic factors (Osborn et al. 1983). The braking phenomenon is itself independent of preserved function of the renal nerves at least in the rat (Petersen and DiBona 1992). It is therefore conceivable that the natriuresis following acute denervation of the kidney may provoke the same intrinsic counterregulatory mechanisms opposing the diuretic effects of denervation over time. If the kidney is reinnervated, dietary sodium restriction increases renal sympathetic nerve activity and contributes to preservation of sodium by an increased proximal reabsorption of sodium. One may conclude that renal denervation impairs the ability of the kidney to conserve sodium during dietary sodium restriction.

In any case, the clinical lesson is that severe restriction of dietary sodium should be avoided in order to avoid negative sodium balance in these patients. Excess dietary sodium should be provided during abnormal enteral or transcutaneous losses of salt or extracellular volume that may be caused by gastroenteritis or hyperthermia. This therapy should necessarily be cautious if there is concurrent cardiac decompensation.

1.2.2.5
Reinnervation of Renal Autografts and Allografts

The transplanted kidney is completely denervated during its transposition from the donor to the recipient. The surgical procedures during autografting of the kidney also imply a complete denervation. However, there is evidence that both renal autografts and renal allografts are not permanently deprived of their nerve supply. Sankari et al. (1992) demonstrated regeneration of both efferent sympathetic renal nerves and of the afferent sympathetic nerves in autotransplanted kidney. The data from their study support the presence of afferent and efferent renal sympathetic nerves, at least 1 year post-transplant.

Reinnervation of the allografted kidney has also been demonstrated both histologically (Gadzar and Dammin 1970,) and by histochemical techniques to localize the catecholamine-containing neural varicosities (Norvell et al. 1969; Nomura et al. 1972). The time frame for the regeneration of renal sympathetic nerves is not firmly established. Gazdar and Dammin (1970) examined the time course and extent of neural degeneration and regeneration in human allografts studied 5 to 3012 days after transplantation. They demonstrated a progressive degeneration of the autonomic renal nerves during the first 3 weeks after transplantation with regeneration beginning at day 28.

In summary, data from animal and human studies clearly demonstrate that transplanted kidneys, whether allografted or autografted, undergo reinnervation. Although the time span for reinnervation may vary in different studies, the start of reinnervation in human transplant allografts is evident as early as 4 weeks following transplantation. Moreover the innervation including renal vasculature, tubular segments and juxtaglomerular apparatus is anatomically indistinguishable from a normal kidney in its native location (DiBona 1987).

However, despite accumulating evidence for a morphological reinnervation of transplanted kidneys, the functional capacity of the reinnervation has been questioned. Hansen et al (1994) examined reflex-induced increase in efferent renal sympathetic nerve activity in response to noradrenaline infusion and lower body negative pressure in transplant patients and in a group of control patients. In patients transplanted more than 27 months previously, a supersensitivity to circulating noradrenaline and a reduced response to lower body negative pressure was found. Rabelink et al. (1993) examined the natriuretic response to head-out water immersion in renal allografted patients 24-56 days after transplantation. The sodium excretion increased equally in transplanted patients and in a group of healthy subjects. Barendregt et al. (1995) studied the effect of different sodium intake in eight recipient and donor pairs. They showed that sodium balance at the low and the high sodium intake periods was not different in the donors and the recipients. In canine kidney Sankari et al. (1992) demonstrated functional afferent renal nerves 12 months after autotransplantation, as assessed by blood pressure response to intrarenal capsaicin injection. It is therefore likely that the morphological reinnervation of transplanted kidneys to a large extent also corresponds to restored function in the renal sympathetic nerves.

1.2.3
Adaptive Changes in the Autotransplanted Kidney

Adaptive changes in the autotransplanted kidney may be both hemodynamic and tubular. They may be both functional and structural in nature. Evidently, early changes comprise functional changes whereas long-term alterations may also be structural in nature.

Early adaptive increase in renal blood flow, glomerular filtration rate, and tubular reabsorption were recognized long ago following a sudden loss of function of the contralateral kidney (Tabei et al. 1983; Potter et al. 1974). We have reported similar hemodynamic and tubular adaptive responses in living kidney donors 1 week after donor nephrectomy (Holdaas et al. 1988). Other more recent observations in kidney donors confirm a short-term response of from 1 to 4 weeks, comprising an increase of renal blood flow and glomerular filtration rate of about 30% in man (ter Wee et al. 1994; Bock et al. 1991). However, this early adaptive response of a remaining healthy native kidney is also seen in the allotransplanted kidney. Actually the denervated renal allograft of seven recipients yielded the same degree of hyperfiltration as its paired remaining donor kidney within the first 24 h following transplantation (Hartmann et al. 1993). The adaptive changes are related to the increased excretory burden of the unpaired kidney. This early response may in part be caused by a reduction in sympathetic efferent renal nerve activity either caused by denervation or by a reduction of intrinsic sympathetic activity on the kidney. Nevertheless the effect of abolishing the renal nerve traffic cannot account for such a major impact on renal function as discussed above. Consequently, adaptive changes would occur in a single functioning autotransplanted kidney, but not if the kidney in situ is functioning normally. The same principle concerns the long-term adaptive process that may solely be regarded as a structural response to the increased functional challenge (analogous to left ventricular hypertrophy associated with hypertension).

1.2.3.1
Increments in Renal Function over Time

If autotransplantation of one kidney takes place and the other kidney is abandoned during the surgical procedure, for example as a result of major aortic and renovascular surgery, long-term adaptive changes over time probably occur in the autotransplanted kidney. Autotransplantation of a solitary functioning kidney is not likely to reveal adaptive changes since a single functioning kidney has already developed these changes (Potter et al. 1974; Tabei et al. 1983; Holdaas et al. 1988; Bock et al. 1991; ter Wee et al. 1994). Since the requirements for development of adaptive changes are not usually fulfilled during renal autotransplantation, the long-term adaptive changes will only briefly be summarized. Lessons from renal allografting are probably relevant to renal autografting. Immunosuppressive and especially cyclosporine treatment would, if anything, ameliorate the adaptive responses. In summary, the changes consist of renal hypertrophy and reinnervation as discussed above. The early increments observed within a week comprise by far the greatest part of the increments in renal blood flow and glomerular filtration rate observed at a later stage. The final increment is usually reached within a month (ter Wee et al. 1994; Flanigan et al. 1968).

1.2.3.2
Renal Functional Reserve

Renal functional reserve defines the ability of the human kidney to increase its glomerular filtration rate over hours following an intake of a protein load (ter Wee et al. 1994; Cassidy and Beck 1988). The functional importance of this phenomenon in man remains questionable. Such a reserve however, as part of a normal physiological in vivo response, may represent a "buffer" against deterioration of kidney function. Renal functional reserve has been thoroughly examined in individuals with a single kidney, such as in kidney donors, uninephrectomized patients with kidney disease, and renal allografted patients (ter Wee et al. 1994; Cassidy and Beck 1988; Hartmann et al. 1994). These studies have unequivocally shown that patients with a single functioning kidney have maintained the ability to increase their glomerular filtration rate following a protein challenge even years after nephrectomy (Cassidy and Beck 1988; ter Wee et al. 1994; Hartmann et al. 1994). Likewise the reabsorptive capacity for sodium may be stimulated by protein ingestion in renal allografted patients (Hartmann et al. 1994). These findings may also be relevant to renal autotransplantation.

1.2.3.3
Progressive Renal Failure Following Major Parenchymal Ablation

Hyperfiltration of remaining nephrons as seen following uninephrectomy (Tabei et al. 1983; Potter et al. 1974; Holdaas et al. 1988; ter Wee et al. 1994; Bock et al. 1991) may be regarded as beneficial because it compensates for the partial loss of kidney function. However, experimental studies both in rats and dogs have clearly shown that hyperfiltration of remaining nephrons following extensive ablation of renal tissue is harmful and may lead to progressive renal failure due to development of progressive glomerular sclerosis (Hostetter et al. 1981; Bourgoignie et al. 1987). In the classical experimental renal ablation model, rats are uninephrecromized and two thirds of the remaining kidney excised, leaving only one sixth of the functional renal mass (Hostetter et al. 1981). The relevance of such experiments in humans may be questioned. Although single reports on progressive renal failure due to sclerosis in single uninephrectomized patients have been presented (Solomon et al. 1985), uninephrectomy with a 50% reduction of renal mass in a large series of patients does not lead to progressive renal disease, either following donor nephrectomy (Talseth et al. 1986; Najarian et al. 1992) or nephrectomy for other reasons. This holds true even decades after the procedure (Foster et al. 1991; Narkun-Burgess et al. 1993).

It may well be that a threshold of hyperfiltration must be reached before the growth process is somehow pushed out of control, leading to progressive damage of remaining kidney tissue. The magnitude of renal mass ablation that can be performed in man without reaching this level is not known. A case of progressive renal failure probably caused by hyperfiltration has been presented in a patient undergoing five-sixth renal ablation (Stahl et al. 1988). However, in a 5 to 17 year follow-up study of 14 patients with a solitary kidney who underwent partial renal ablation corresponding to a remaining renal mass of only one eighth to three eighths of normal, only two patients revealed progression to renal end-stage failure. The other twelve patients maintained a stable serum creatinine level. The patients were, however, at high risk of developing proteinuria and glomerulopathy and were considered at risk of future impairment of renal function (Barajas et al. 1984).

Vigorous treatment of concurrent hypertension is advocated in patients to help avoid loss of kidney function (Foster et al. 1991; Raine 1994). There is an ongoing discussion whether ACE inhibitors may exert a higher level of nephroprotection than other antihypertensive drugs in these patients, as has been shown for early diabetic nephropathy, a disease also characterized by a state of glomerular hyperfiltration (Viberti et al. 1994). Recent data show that ACE inhibitors have outstanding renoprotective effects in nondiabetic kidney disease of different origin (Maschio et al. 1996).

In patients with a normally functioning kidney alongside of a partially ablated and autotransplanted kidney, the hyperfiltration will (as previously discussed) be less pronounced. A functioning remaining kidney may therefore represent a protection against "hyperfiltration parenchymal damage" in a partially ablated and autotransplanted kidney. Obviously, in any case, limitation of the resection is warranted in order to obtain the optimal function of the graft. The magnitude of tissue resection has to be a compromise between the need for radical surgery and the prospects for future function in the autograft as discussed elsewhere in this book.

References

Barajas L (1978) Innervation of the renal cortex. Fed Proc 37:192-201

Barajas L, Powers K, Wang P (1984) Innervation of the renal cortical tubules: a quantitative study. Am J Physiol 247:F50-F60

Barajas L, Liu L, Powers K (1992) Anatomy of the renal innervation: intrarenal aspects and ganglia of origin. Can J Physiol Pharmacol 70:735-49

Barendregt JNM, van Nispen tot Pannerden LLAM, Chang PC (1995) Interactions between sodium balance, intrarenal dopamine synthesis, and sympathetic activity in HLA-identical kidney donors and recipients Nephrol Dial Transplant 10:341-348

Bell GM, Reid J, Buist TAS (1987) Percutaneous transluminal angioplasty improves blood pressure and renal function in renovascular hypertension. Quart J Med. 63:393-403

Blake WD (1962) Relative roles of glomerular filtration and tubular reabsorption in denervation diuresis. Am J Phys 202:777-783

Blaufox MD, Lewis EJ, Jagger P, Lauler D, Hickler R, Merill JP (1969) Physiologic responses of the transplanted human kidney. New Engl J Med 289:62-66

Bock HA, Gregor M, Huser B, Rist M, Landmann J, Thiel G (1991) Glomerulare Hyperfiltration nach unilateraler Nephrektomie bei Gesunden. Schweiz Med Wochenschr 121:1835-1835

Bourgoignie JJ, Gavellas G, Martinez E et al. (1987) Glomerular function and morphology after renal mass reduction in dogs. Lab Clin Med 109:380-388

Bricker NS, Guild WR, Reardan JB, Merill JP (1956) Studies on the functional capacity of a denervated homotransplanted kidney in an identical twin with parallel observations in the donor. J Clin Invest 35:364-380

Bubeck B (1995) Radionuclide techniques for the evaluation of renal function: advantages over conventional methoology. Curr Opin Nephrol Hypertens 4:514-519

Cassidy MJD, Beck RM (1988) Renal functional reserve in living related kidney donors. Am J Kidney Dis 11:468-472

Dean RH, Kieffer RW, Smith BM (1968) Renovascular hypertension: anatomical and renal function changes during drug therapy. Arch Surg 116:1408-15

Dean RH, Tribble RW, Hansen KJ, O'Neil E, Craven TE, Redding JF (1991) Evolution of renal insufficiency in ischemic nephropathy. Ann Surg 213:446-55

DiBona GF (1987) Renal innervation and denervation: Lessons from renal transplantation reconsidered. Artif Organs 11:457-462

Eyler WR, Clark ND, Garman JF (1962) Angiography of the renal areas including a comparative study of renal arterial stenosis in patients with and without hypertension. Radiology 78:879-92

Ferguson M, Bell C (1988) Ultrastructural localization and characterization of sensory nerves in the rat kidney. J Comp Neurol 274:9-16

Flanigan WJ, Burns RO, Takacs FJ, Merill JP (1968) Serial studies of glomerular filtration rate and renal plasma flow in kidney transplant donors, identical twins and allograft recipients. Am J Surg 116:788-794

Foster MH, Sant GR, Donohoe JF, Harrington JT (1991) Prolonged survival with a remnant kidney. Am J Kidney Dis 17:261-165

Gazdar AF, Dammin GJ (1970) Neural degeneration and regeneration in human renal transplants. N Engl J Med 238:222-224

Gill JR, Barter FC (1966) Adrenergic nervous system in sodium metabolism. II. Effects of guanethidine on the renal response to sodium deprivation in normal man. N Engl J Med 275:1466-1471

Goldblatt H, Lynch J, Hanzal RF, Summerville WW (1934) Studies on experimental hypertension. I. The production of persistent elevation of systolic blood pressure by means of renal ischaemia. J Exptl Med 59:347

Grandjean B, Annat G, Vincent M, Sassard J (1978) Influence of renal nerves on renin secretion in the conscious dog. Pflügers Arch 373:161-165

Greenberg SG, Tershner S, Osborn JL (1991) Neurogenic regulation of rate of achieving sodium balance after increasing sodium intake. Am J Physiol 261:F300- F307

Hansen JM, Abilgaard U, Fogh-Andersen N, Kanstrup IL, Bratholm P, Plum I, Strandgaard S (1994) The transplanted human kidney does not achieve functional reinnervation. Clin Sci 87:13-20

Harkonen S, Kjellstrand C (1981) Contrast nephropathy. Am J Nephrol 1:69-77

Hartmann A, Bugge J, Osnes S, Stenstrøm J, Bentdal Ø, Berg KJ, Fauchald P, Holdaas H (1993) Immediate and early function of living donor grafts as compared to the remaining donor kidneys. J Amer Soc Nephrol 4:939

Hartmann A, Nilssen HL, Draganov B, Holdaas H, Bentdal Ø, Berg KJ (1994) Renal reserve is present several years following donor nephrectomy. J Amer Soc Nephrol 5:1011

Heyeraas KJ, Aukland K (1987) Interlobular arterial resistance: influence of renal arterial pressure and angiotensin II. Kidney Int 33:1291-1298

Holdaas H, Langård Ø, Eide I, Kiil F (1981a) Mechanism of renin release during renal nerve stimulation in dogs. Scand J Clin Lab Invest 41:617-625

Holdaas H, DiBona GF, Kiil F (1981b) Effect of low level renal nerve stimulation on renin release from nonfiltering kidneys. Am J Physiol 241:F156-F161

Holdaas H, DiBona GF (1981) The role of left atrial receptors in the regulation of renin release in anesthetized dogs. Acta Physiol Scand 11:497-500

Holdaas H, DiBona GF (1984) On the existence of renal vasodilator nerves. Proc Soc Exp Biol 176:426-433

Holdaas H, Hartmann A, Talseth T, Berg KJ, Fauchald P, Stenstrøm J, Djøseland O, Nordal KP, Brodwall E (1988) Short-term changes in renal function of the remaining kidney after donor nephrectomy. Transplant Proc 20:434-435

Hollenberg NK, Adams DF, Solomon H, et al. (1975) Renal vascular tone in essential and secondary hypertension. Medicine 564:29-44

Holley KE, Hunt JC, Brown AL, et al. (1964) Renal artery stenosis: a clinical pathologic study in normotensive and hypertensive patients. Am J Med 37:14-22

Hostetter TH, Olson JL, Rennke HG et al. (1981) Hyperfiltration in remnant nephrons: a potentially adverse response to renal ablation. Am J Physiol 245:F85- F93

Kasiske BL (1987) Possible causes and consequences of hypertension in stable renal transplant patients. Transplantation 44:639

Knuepfer MM, Schramm LP (1987) The conduction velocities and spinal projections of single renal afferent fibres in the rat. Brain Res 435:167-173

Kopp U, Holdaas H, DiBona GF (1984) Neural regulation of renal function: Sodium excretion and renin release. In: Kotchen TA, Guthrie GP Jr (eds) Hypertension and the Brain. pp 113-126

Kopp UC, DiBona GF (1992) The neural control of renal function. In Seldin DW, Giebisch G (eds): The kidney: physiology and pathophysiology, 2nd edn. Raven, New York, pp 1157-1204

Langård Ø, Holdaas H, Eide I, Kiil F (1981) Conditions for humoral a-adrenoceptor stimulation of renin release in anesthetized dogs. Scand J Clin Lab Invest 41:527-534

Lüscher TF, Kaplan NM (1992) Renovascular and renal parenchymatous hypertension. Springer Verlag, Berlin Heidelberg New York.

Martin LG, Casarella WJ, Gaylord GM (1987) Azotemia caused by renal artery stenosis: treatment by percutaneous angioplasty. Am J Radiol 150:839-844

Maschio G, Alberti D, Janin G, Locatelli F, Mann JFE, Motolese M, Ponticelli C, Ritz E, Zucchelli P, The Angiotensin-Converting-Enzyme Inhibition in Progressive Renal Insufficiency Study Group (1996) Effect of the angiotensin-converting-enzyme inhibitor benazepril on the progression of chronic renal insufficiency. N Engl J Med 334:939-945

Miller WL, Thomas RA, Berner RM, Rubio R (1978) Adenosine production in the ischemic kidney. Circ Res 43:390-397

Mitchell GAG (1950) The nerve supply of the kidneys. Acta Anat 10:1-37

Moss NG (1989) Electrophysiological characteristics of renal sensory receptors and afferent renal nerves. Miner Electrolyte Metab 15:59-65

Najarian JS, Chavers BM Talseth, McHugh LE, Matas AJ (1992) 20 years or more of follow-up of living kidney donors. Lancet 340:807-810

Narkun-Burgess DM, Nolan CR, Norman JE, Page WF, Miller PL, Meyer TW (1993) Forty-five year follow-up after nephrectomy. Kidney Int 43:1110-1115

Nomura G, Kurosaki M, Katabatake T, Kibe Y, Takeuchi J (1972) Reinnervation and renin release after unilateral renal denervation in the dog. J Appl Physiol 33:649-655

Norvell JE, Weitsen HA, Dwyer JJ (1969) Degeneration and regeneration of adrenergic nerves in the autotransplanted kidney. Transplantation 7:218-220

Novick AC (1991). Management of renovascular disease. A surgical perspective. Circulation 83[2 Suppl I]:167-171

Novick AC, Gephardt G, Guz B, Steinmuller D, Tubbs RR (1991) Long-term follow-up after partial removal of a solitary kidney. N Engl J Med 325:1058-1062

Osborn JL, Holdaas H, Thames MD, Di Bona GF (1983) Renal adrenoceptor modification of antinatriuretic and renin secretion responses to low level nerve stimulation in the dog. Circulation Res 53:298-305

Pattynama PM, Becker GJ, Brown J, Zemel G, Benenati JF, Katzen BT (1994) Percutaneous angioplasty for atherosclerotic renal artery disease: effect on renal function in azotemic patients. Cardiovasc Intervent Radiol 18:143-146

Paulsen D, Klöw NE, Rogstad B, Lien B, Vatne K, Fauchald P (1996) 419 patients treated by percutaneous transluminal renal angioplasty (PTRA). Abstract XXXIIIrd Congress of the European Renal Association p 60

Pedersen EB (1994) Angiotensin converting enzyme inhibitor renography. Pathophysiological, diagnostic and therapeutic aspects in renal artery stenosis. Nephrol Dial Transplant 9:482-492

Petersen J, DiBona GF (1992) Effects of renal denervation on sodium balance and renal function during chronic furosemide administration in rats. J Pharm Exptl Ther 262:1103-1109

Peterson TV, Benjamin BA, Hurst NL, Euler CG (1991) Renal nerves and postprandial renal excretion in the conscious monkey. Am J Physiol 261:R1197-R1203

Pickering TG (1991) Diagnosis and evaluation of renovascular hypertension. Indications for therapy. Circulation 83[2 Suppl]:147-154

Pohl MA, Horner C, Goormastic M, et al. (1991) Does renal revascularization preserve renal function in patients with atherosclerotic renal artery stenosis? An ongoing prospective study. J Am Soc Nephrol 2:242

Pohl MA (1993) The ischemic kidney and hypertension. Am J Kidney Dis 21[Suppl 2]:22-28

Potter DE, Leumann EP, Sakai T, Holliday MA (1974) Early responses of glomerular filtration rate to unilateral nephrectomy. Kidney Int 5:131-136

Pyøræelæ K, De Backer G, Graham I, on behalf of the Task Force (1994) Prevention of coronary heart disease in clinical practice. Recommendations of the Task Force of the European Society of Cardiology, European Atherosclerosis Society and European Society of Hypertension. Eur Heart J 15:1300-1333

Rabelink TJ, van Tilborg KA, Hené J, Koomans HA (1993) Natriuretic response to head-out immersion in humans with recent kidney transplants. Clin Sci 85:471-477

Raine AEG (1994) Hypertension and the kidney. Br Med Bull 50:322-341

Rosenthal T (1993) Drug therapy of renovascular hypertension. Drugs 45:895-909

Sadowski J, Kurkus J, Gellert R (1979) Denervated and intact kidney response to saline load in awake and anesthetized dogs. Am J Physiol 237:F262-F267

Sankari B, Stowe N, Gavin JP, Satoh S, Nally JV, Novick AC (1992) Studies on the afferent and efferent nerves following autotransplantation of the canine kidney. J Urol 148:206-210

Schefft P, Novick AC, Stewart BH, Straffon RH (1980) Renal revascularization in patients with total occlusion of the renal artery. J Urol 124:184-186

Schreiber MJ, Pohl MA, Novick AC (1984) The natural history of atherosclerotic and fibrous renal artery disease. Urol Clin North Am 11:383-392

Scoble JE, Hamilton G (1990) Atherosclerotic renovascular disease. Remediable cause of renal failure in the elderly. BMJ 300:1670-1671

Setaro JF, Chen CC, Hoffer PB, et al. (1991) Captopril renography in the diagnosis of renal artery stenosis and the prediction of improvement with revascularization. The Yale vascular center experience. Am J Hypertens 4:S698-S705

Sfakianakis GN, Bourgoignie JJ, Jaffe D, et al. (1987) Single dose captopril scintigraphy in the diagnosis of renovascular hypertension. J Nucl Med 28:1383-1392

Solomon LR, Mallick NP, Lawler W (1985) Progressive renal failure in a remnant kidney. BMJ 291:1610-1611

Sos TA (1991) Angioplasty for the treatment of azotemia and renovascular hypertension in atherosclerotic renal artery disease. Circulation 83[2 Suppl]:162-166

Stahl PA, Low I, Schoeppe W (1988) Progressive renal failure in a patient after one and two-thirds nephrectomy. Klin Wochenschr 66:508-510

Svetkey LP, Wilkinson R, Dunnick NR, et al. (1991) Captopril renography in the diagnosis of renovascular hypertension. Am J Hypertens 4:S711-S715

Tabei K, Levenson DJ, Brenner BM (1983) Early enhancement of fluid transport in rabbit proximal straight tubules after loss of contralateral renal excretory function. J. Clin Invest 72:871-881

Talseth T, Fauchald P, Skrede S, Djøseland O, Berg KJ, Stenstrøm J, Heilo A, Brodwall EK, Flatmark A (1986) Long-term blood pressure and renal function in kidney donors. Kidney Int 29:1072-1076

ter Wee PM, Tegzess AM, Donker AJ (1994) Pair-tested renal reserve filtration capacity in kidney recipients and their donors. J Am Soc Nephrol 4:1798-1808

Textor SC (1994) Renovascular hypertension. Endocrinol Metab Clin North Am 23:235-253

Thames MD, DiBona GF (1979) Renal nerves modulate the secretion of renin mediated by non-neural mechanisms. Circ Res 44:645-652

The Scandinavian simvastatin survival study group (1994) Randomised trial of cholesterol lowering in 4444 patients with coronary heart disease: the Scandinavian simvastatin survival study. Lancet 344:1383-1389

Viberti G, Mogensen CE, Groop LC, Pauls JF, for the European Microalbuminuria Captopril Study Group (1994) Effect of captopril on progression to clinical proteinuria in patients with insulin-dependent diabetes mellitus and microalbuminuria. JAMA 271:275-279

Wilcox CS, Aminoff MJ, Slater JDH (1977) Sodium homeostasis in patients with autonomic failure. Clin Sci 53:321-32

Radiological Investigation and Interventional Procedures in Patients with Renal Artery Disease

Nils Einar Kløw and Karleif Vatne

2.1
Introduction

Atherosclerosis and fibromuscular dysplasia (FMD) are the two most common causes of renal artery stenoses and aneurysms, while Takayasu's arteritis is a frequent cause of arterial stenosis in persons from Asia. Renal artery FMD is usually identified by its characteristic angiographic appearance and typical location in the nonorificial part of the renal arterial tree. In most patients with atherosclerotic renal artery disease, atherosclerotic changes can also be seen in the lumbar aorta and the iliac arteries.

A renal artery lesion represents a threat to the patient, through its potential for causing renovascular hypertension, renal failure, or serious hemorrhage from aneurysm rupture. The anatomical lesion responsible can usually be corrected and should thus be diagnosed and treated to cure or improve renovascular hypertension and to preserve or improve renal function before irreversible damage has been established.

Intraarterial renal angiography has been the only reliable method for diagnosing renal artery abnormalities. During the past 10 years, several new, less invasive methods have evolved to compete with conventional angiography. Further development is expected within the next few years which will result in a change from invasive to noninvasive investigation.

Percutaneous transluminal renal angioplasty (PTRA) and surgery are both options for active management of renal artery stenoses (Novick et al. 1987; Weibull et al. 1993; Soulen 1994), but PTRA has increasingly replaced surgery since its introduction in 1978 (Grüntzig et al. 1978). The introduction of stents has further improved this technique (Palmaz et al. 1987; Dorros et al. 1993).

The results of PTRA are excellent in stenoses caused by FMD (Tegtmeyer et al. 1991). In atherosclerotic lesions, the primary technical success rates are high, but longer term results are vitiated by recurrent stenoses (Weibull et al. 1993; Jensen et al 1995). Surgery is still the method of choice for renal artery aneurysms, for stenoses unsuitable for PTRA, and when previous PTRAs have been unsuccessful.

2.2
Screening Methods

Renovascular hypertension is diagnosed in 1%-5% of the general hypertensive population (see Chap. 1). This low prevalence, combined with the fact that there is no simple and entirely reliable screening method available, makes it inappropriate to recommend screening of all hypertensive patients for renal artery disease. However, it is possible to identify subgroups of patients in whom there is increased probability of renovascular hypertension. These subgroups include young women and groups of individuals with one or more of the following features: the onset of hypertension before the age of 30 or after 50, abrupt onset of symptoms, negative family history, malignant hypertension, and development of azotemia during the use of ACE inhibitors (Pickering 1991).

Screening tests, such as the oral captopril test, captopril renography, selective catheterization of the renal veins for renin determination, and duplex Doppler imaging (see Chap. 1) may be used to select patients for further investigation. Various angiographic examinations such as intravenous digital subtraction angiography, magnetic resonance angiography, and spiral computed tomographic angiography can be performed on outpatients. However, intraarterial renal angiography is still the gold standard for detection of renal artery disease. Some of the other angiographic techniques may replace conventional angiography in the near future.

2.3
Preoperative Investigation

The radiological investigation preceding interventional therapy for renal artery lesions includes angiography of both the renal and the iliac arteries. The angiogram should aim to detect accessory arteries as well as any abnormalities in the main renal arteries and branches. Any abnormality in the iliac arteries should be identified to aid in determining the reimplantation site when autotransplantation is planned.

A renal artery lumen diameter reduction of at least 50% is supposed to be required to cause hypertension. However, the exact reduction is often difficult to determine due to diffuse lesions, poststenotic dilatation, and suboptimal projection. Measurement of the transstenotic pressure gradient is a useful supplementary tool in such cases (Schmitz-Rode et al. 1993; Kløw and Vatne 1994).

2.3.1
Arteriography

The arteriographic investigation includes the injection of an intraarterial contrast medium. Using small diameter catheters, the angiography can be performed on an outpatient basis in selected patients. A high-quality angiogram can be obtained using a film exchanger, digital subtraction, or cinefilm.

2.3.1.1
Renal Arteries

The contrast medium should be injected into the abdominal aorta at the origin of the renal arteries to avoid the superimposition of the mesenteric branches on the renal arteries. We recommend a midstream injection through a "tennis racket" or "pigtail" catheter with multiple sideholes. If possible, selective injection into the renal arteries should be avoided because of the risk of renal artery dissection and occlusion. The frontal view should be supplemented with oblique projections whenever necessary to reveal any ostial lesions or stenoses in bends of the renal arteries.

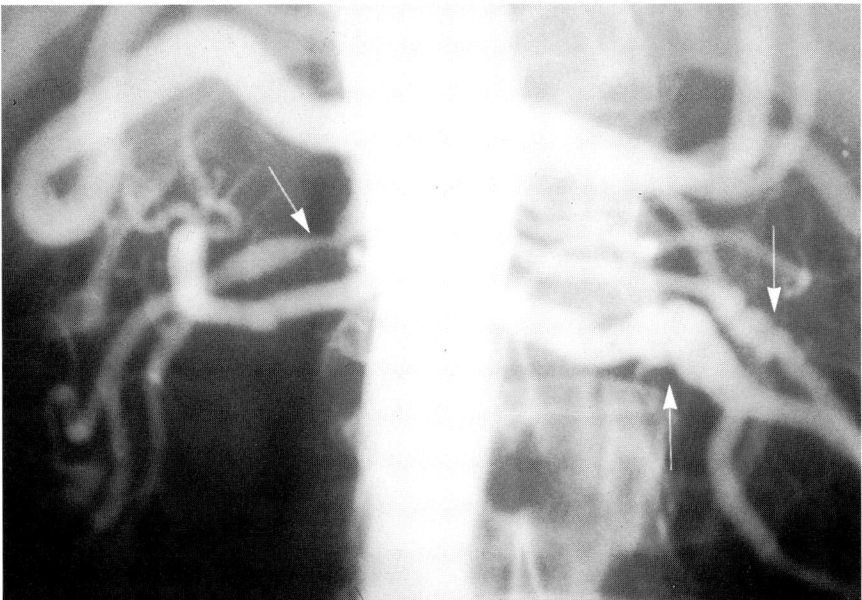

Fig. 2.1. Intraarterial angiographic examination before PTRA in a patient with multiple renal arteries. On the right side a solitary stenosis is present in the most cranial of the two renal arteries (→), and on the left side, lesions typical for fibromuscular dysplasia are seen in both the two renal arteries (→)

Accessory renal arteries are quite common (Kjellevand et al. 1991) and their preoperative visualization is important to avoid damage during surgery and to diagnose any lesion that should be treated (Fig. 2.1). All stenotic arteries must be treated to ensure the optimal result of a revascularization procedure. The angiogram must be of a high quality to detect stenoses of peripheral renal artery branches. It should include images of both the arterial and the parenchymal phases to determine the kidney size and to identify peripheral stenoses or possibly infarcted areas.

Following total occlusion of a renal artery, successful revascularization may be possible, provided extrarenal collaterals have preserved renal parenchyma. The size of the kidney, and an expanded angiographic series to look for possible delayed circulation, will give important information on whether its is worthwhile to attempt treatment.

2.3.1.2
Iliac Arteries

Most patients with atherosclerotic lesions in the renal arteries have generalized atherosclerotic disease also affecting the iliac arteries. Arteriography of the iliac arteries must therefore be performed to detect any stenoses or aneurysms before autotransplantation can be performed (Fig. 2.2).

The angiogram may determine the site for reimplantation, i.e., whether the left or right side or whether the external or internal artery should be chosen for an anastomosis to the renal artery. It may also reveal the need for preparatory vascular surgery.

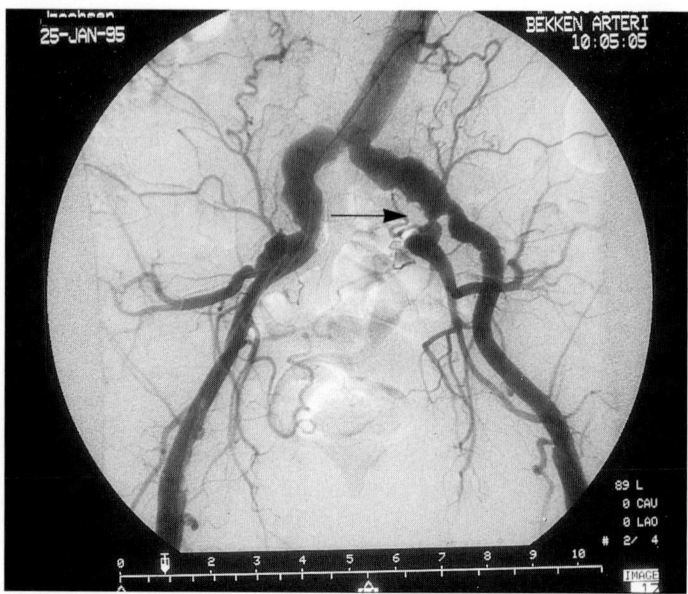

Fig. 2.2. Intraarterial digital subtraction angiography of the iliac arteries showing stenosis of the left internal iliac artery at the bifurcation of the common iliac artery (→), usually precluding anastomosis of the transplant artery to this artery. In this patient aortobifemoral by pass and renal autotransplantation were performed simultaneously

Stenosis of the internal iliac artery at the bifurcation of the common iliac artery is common and may be difficult to identify in a frontal view. A left and right oblique projection at about 60° usually give sufficient information when contrast medium is injected immediately above the aortic bifurcation. The images should include the iliac arteries and the lower lumbar aorta.

2.3.1.3
Contrast Medium

All contrast media may affect renal function and even induce acute renal failure in some patients. The risk of renal failure is related to the volume used. Nevertheless, there should be an adequate number of projections for a complete examination. The risk of renal deterioration is increased in all kinds of nephropathies and in dehydrated patients. Good hydration is important in all patients referred for angiography in order to reduce the nephrotoxic effects of the contrast media. Low osmolar contrast media, such as the nonionic contrast media, affect renal function to a very limited extent (Barrett and Carlisle 1993). One of these contrast media should therefore be used in patients with impaired renal function. Recently, a new generation of isosmolar contrast media, the nonionic dimers (iotrolan, iodixanol), has become available. These new contrast media are supposed to have minimal nephrotoxic effects (Kløw et al. 1993).

2.3.2.
Intravenous Digital Subtraction Angiography

Intravenous digital subtraction angiography can easily be performed in outpatients, causing less inconvenience to the patient than intraarterial angiography. Moreover, the examination can be combined with renal vein renin measurements. However, intravenous angiography is less reliable than intraarterial angiography, since lesions of branch renal arteries are especially likely to be missed (Havey et al. 1985; Katzen 1995).

2.3.3
Magnetic Resonance Angiography

Magnetic resonance angiography includes a class of MR imaging techniques designed to create angiographic images. The techniques are noninvasive and do not require the use of contrast media or ionizing radiation. MR angiography of the renal arteries has proved itself to be less than ideal (Fig. 2.3A). The image quality is inferior to MR angiography of other vessels, such as the carotid arteries, since respiratory motion and aortic pulsation reduce the quality. The sensitivity of these methods for evaluating renal artery stenosis is comparable with i.v. digital subtraction angiography. Lesions of the main renal artery can be detected, but accessory arteries are easily missed and the severity of the stenosis is usually overestimated. However, in transplanted kidneys both the renal artery and branches of the main renal artery can be visualized (Fig. 2.4). In patients with suspected venous thrombosis MR angiography has provided accurate information (Debatin et al. 1991; Smith and Bakke 1993; Krestin 1994).

2.3.4
Computed Tomographic Angiography

The recent introduction of spiral CT angiography has added a new, minimally invasive, technique for detecting renal artery stenoses. To obtain an optimized CT angiogram,

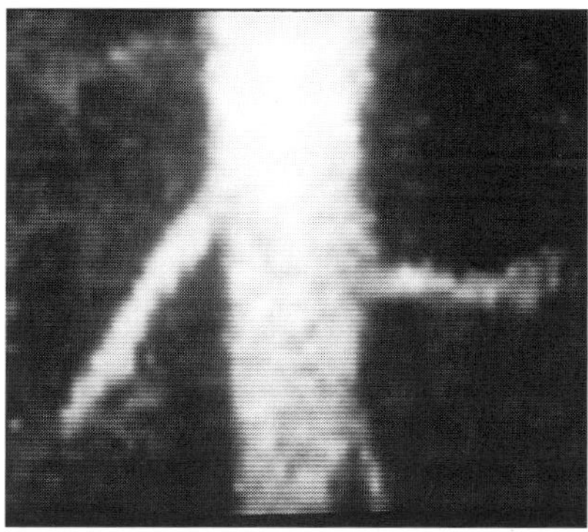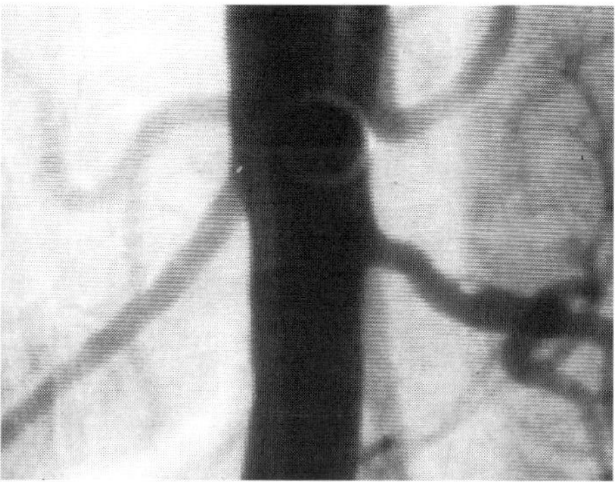

Fig. 2.3A,B. Magnetic resonance (MR) angiography (A) and intraarterial angiography (B) of normal renal arteries in the same patient. The MR angiography only shows the proximal parts of the renal arteries. Three-dimensional time-of-flight MR angiography was used (from Smith et al. 1993 with permission)

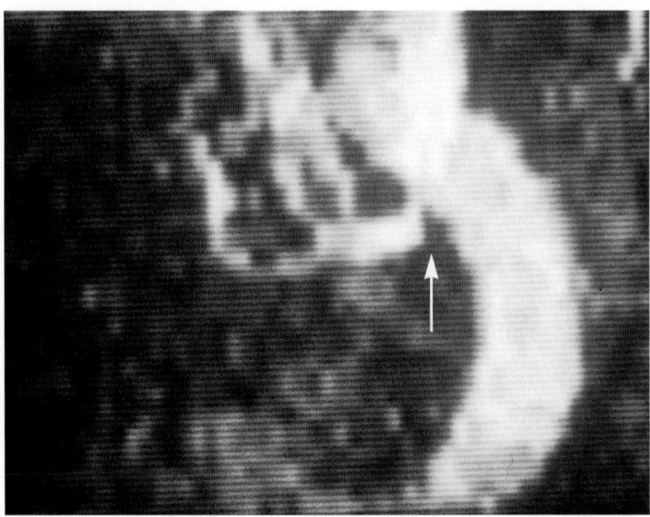

Fig. 2.4. Magnetic resonance (MR) angiography of an autotransplanted kidney in the right iliac fossa. The renal transplant artery has been anastomosed to the internal iliac artery. A stenosis in the area of the anastomosis is demonstrated ($\rightarrow$). Note that also segmental arteries can be demonstrated by MR angiography in this transplanted kidney

the examination requires the cooperation of the patient who must hold his breath for 30 s, while the contrast medium is injected intravenously. The advantage of the volumetric spiral CT acquisition is that three-dimensional renderings are generated which provide views from innumerable angles. Initial results are comparable to the results of MR angiography. Accessory renal arteries are often missed, and an accurate estimation of the degree of stenosis is difficult (Rubin et al. 1995; Bluemke and Chambers 1995).

2.3.5
Duplex Doppler Imaging

The velocity waveforms emanating from the renal arteries can be recorded by duplex Doppler imaging. A number of criteria have been developed for diagnosing renal artery stenosis, such as the ratio of peak systolic velocities in the stenotic segment of the renal artery and the aorta, distal turbulence, and analysis of distal damping with indices such as acceleration time, acceleration index, and resistive index. The examination may be technically unsatisfactory in up to 40% of in situ kidneys. Adequate examination of stenotic segments can usually only be obtained from the proximal end of the renal artery and accessory renal arteries are often overlooked. On the other hand, duplex sonography appears to be a reliable, noninvasive method for evaluating arterial stenosis following renal transplantation (Snider et al. 1989; Kliewer et al. 1993; Saarinen et al. 1994; Schwerk et al. 1994).

2.4
Postoperative Investigations

Autotransplantation is the principal procedure for the surgical management of renal artery stenoses at our hospital (Flatmark et al. 1989; Brekke et al. 1992). The kidney is reimplanted to the iliac fossa (Fig. 2.5) with the renal artery anastomosed to the internal or external iliac artery (Fig. 2.6). Urinary continuity is reestablished by ureteroneocystostomy (Fig. 2.7).

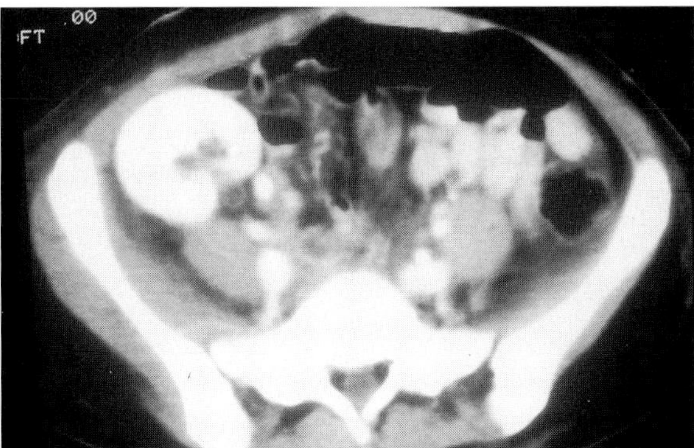

Fig. 2.5. Renal autotransplantation into the left iliac fossa. The axial computed tomographic examination after intravenous contrast medium injection shows the superficial position of the kidney, in front of the psoas muscle and close to the abdominal wall

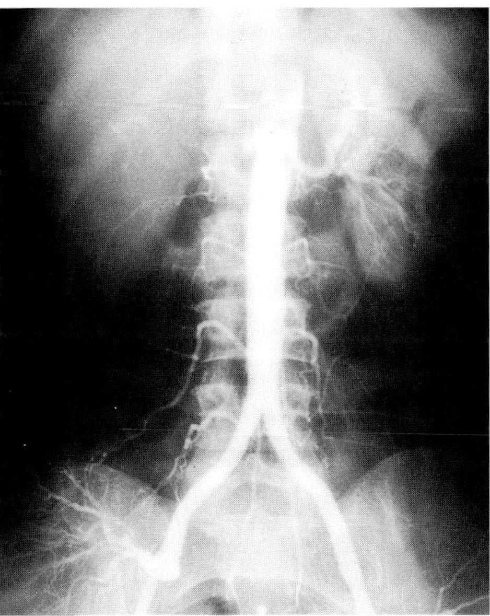

Fig. 2.6. Renal autotransplantation of the right kidney into the right iliac fossa. The intraarterial angiographic examination shows the occluded (ligated) right renal artery and the transplant artery anastomosed to the internal iliac artery

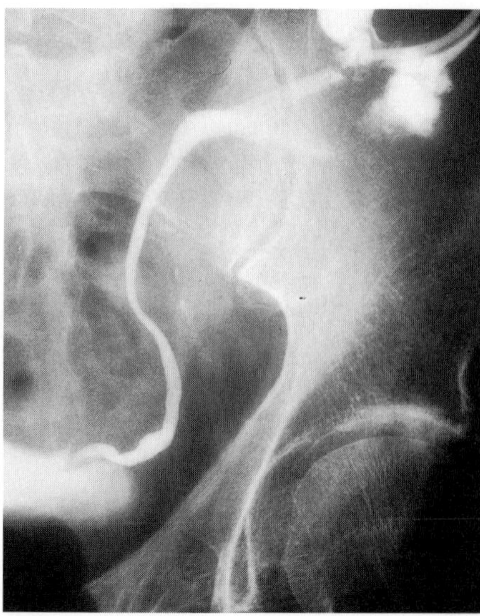

Fig. 2.7. Renal autotransplantation into the left iliac fossa. The antegrade pyelogram shows the ureter reimplanted into the urinary bladder. Free passage of the contrast medium without any leakage

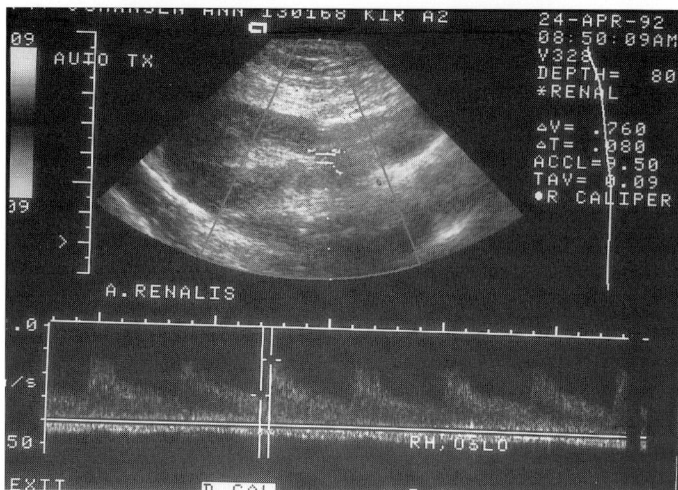

Fig. 2.8. Duplex Doppler sonography of a renal autotransplant. The spectral Doppler curve in the lower part shows increased peak systolic velocity, to about 1.5 m/s, indicating an artery stenosis. Angiographically, the stenosis was significant, and treated with balloon angioplasty 65 days after transplantation

Vascular postoperative complications include renal artery and vein thrombosis. Since duplex sonography appears to be a reliable initial, noninvasive method of evaluating these complications, we routinely examine patients at the end of the first postoperative week to assess the circulation of the graft and the flow in the renal artery and vein (Fig. 2.8). Angiography is performed when vascular complications are suspected clinically or during duplex sonography.

Other postoperative routines include investigations to check the drainage of urine, to exclude urine leakage, and hematoma or lymphocele formation (Fig. 2.9). In most patients, urinary drainage and possible complications can be evaluated by sonography (Fig. 2.10) in combination with duplex sonography. In some patients urography or pyelography is indicated for evaluation of urinary flow or to detect urine leakage or fistula formation.

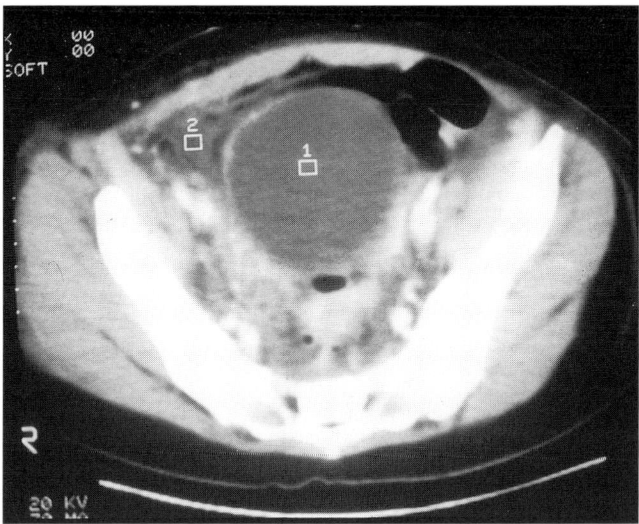

FFig. 2.9. Small lymphocele (2) lateral to the urinary bladder (1) demonstrated by computed tomographic examination. The lymphocele consists of fluid with low attenuation. Measurements in this patients showed attenuation between -5 and -21 Hounsfield units in the lymphocele and +5 in the bladder

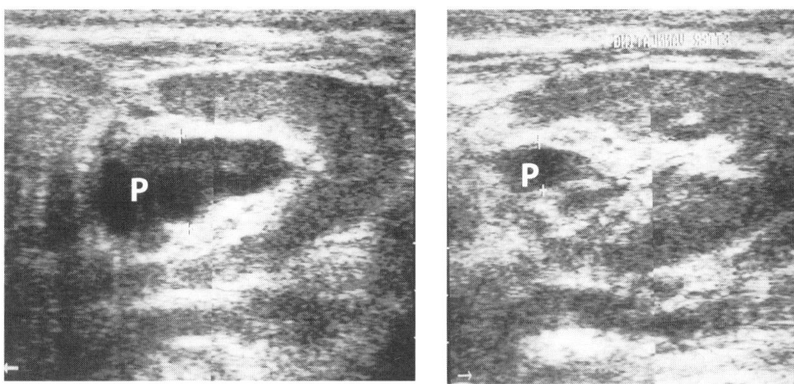

Fig. 2.10 A,B. Sonography of an autotransplanted kidney 8 days after transplantation. Sonogram A shows dilatation of the renal pelvis (P). Sonogram B was made after bladder emptying, showing only a slightly dilated pelvis. This demonstrates the importance of an empty bladder during the examination whenever the size of the renal pelvis is evaluated in kidney transplants

Early stenosis in a transplant artery usually occurs at the site of, or near to, the anastomosis, and may be caused by inadequate surgical technique, the formation of an intimal crest, or arterial kinking (Frauchiger et al. 1994). These complications may cause early graft dysfunction, worsening of a preexistent hypertension, or de novo hypertension. Furthermore, patients treated for renal artery stenosis are at an increased risk of developing new stenoses at any time after the transplant (Tollefson and Ernst 1991). Clinically suspected arterial stenosis should be verified by arteriography which should include both the renal transplant and any in situ kidney.

2.5
Percutaneous Transluminal Renal Angioplasty

Since the introduction of renal angioplasty by Grüntzig in 1978 (Grüntzig et al. 1978), the technique has been further developed and PTRA has become the primary and definitive treatment of renal artery stenosis in most patients. PTRA was introduced in our department in 1982. Figure 2.11 shows the number of patients treated for renal artery stenosis with PTRA or autotransplantation from 1982 to 1992. Additional patients underwent autotransplantation for renal artery aneurysms. Note that PTRA was attempted in some of the patients before autotransplantation. Also, some patients referred for PTRA were treated for stenosis of the autotransplant artery. Some PTRAs were performed on the in situ kidney in patients previously treated with unilateral autotransplantation.

Guide catheter assisted angioplasty is used in our department (Fig. 2.12). An 8F or 9F guide catheter is advanced to the ostium of the renal artery to be dilated. A guide wire and balloon catheter are advanced through the guide catheter to the renal ostium. Following this, the 0.014 in. angioplasty guide wire is advanced across the stenosis, and the low profile balloon catheter is advanced over the guide wire into the lesion. Using this technique, contrast medium can be injected for accurate positioning of the balloon, and the transstenotic pressure gradient can be measured. The double-guide wire technique is easy to perform, and the additional support is useful for passing tight stenoses. The limitation of this technique lies in the need for large arterial sheaths

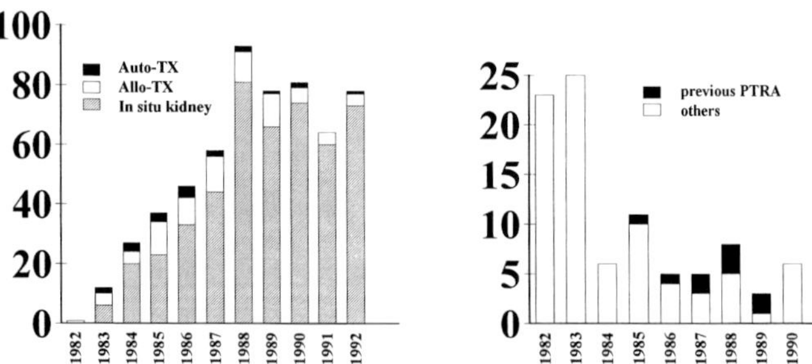

Fig. 2.11. The left panel shows the number of percutaneous transluminal renal angioplasties (PTRAs) performed at our hospital from 1982 to 1992, of in situ kidneys, allotransplanted and autotransplanted kidneys. The right panel shows the number of autotransplantations for renal artery stenosis performed at our hospital in the same time period. The filled bars indicate the number of patients with previously attempted PTRA

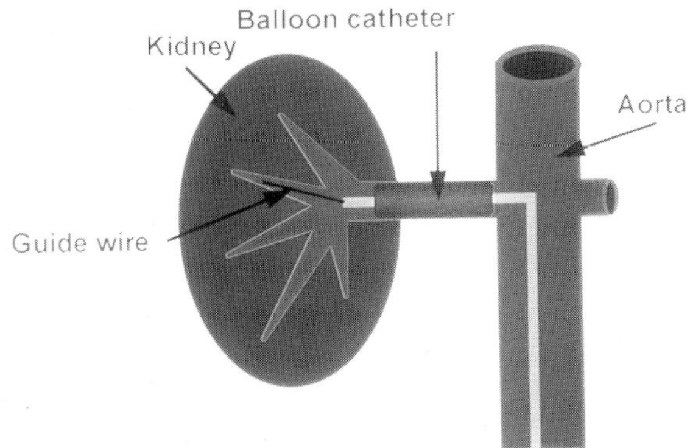

Fig. 2.12. Percutaneous transluminal renal angioplasty using a guide catheter. The tip of the guide catheter is positioned in the ostium of the renal artery and left in place during the whole procedure. The guide wire and the balloon are advanced into the stenosis through the guide catheter (from Kløw and Vatne 1994)

(8–9F), and a balloon which must be less than 8 mm (White et al. 1991; Korogi and Takahashi 1993; Kløw and Vatne 1994).

PTRA is technically demanding, requiring a highly skilled operator to obtain good results in complex lesions. The availability of urgent surgery services for kidney salvage is important if the PTRA is complicated by acute arterial occlusion. Improvements in the treatment of the more complex stenoses include hydrophilic, low-profile high-pressure balloon catheters, soft and steerable tips to the guide wires, the guide catheter technique, and the placement of stents (Palmaz et al. 1987). All of these have improved the technical success rate in treatment of ostial stenoses, stenoses in segmental arteries and at bifurcations, asymmetric stenoses, and stenoses in patients with lumbar aortic disease. However, patients with a lumbar aortic aneurysm or occlusive disease with renal artery involvement should be considered for surgery (Fig. 2.13).

We have recently reviewed all patients who underwent PTRA between 1982 and 1992. There were 595 PTRA procedures performed on a total of 419 patients. Successful results, as judged by the primary angiogram, were achieved in 92% of the patients treated (technical success rate) and another 3.5% were improved. At final angiographic follow-up after one, or up to six, angioplasties, successful treatment was achieved in 83% and improvement in another 7% of the patients. In three patients the kidney was successfully autotransplanted after acute renal artery occlusion, and in one patient the kidney was autotransplanted the next day following an unsuccessful PTRA. Another 12 patients underwent autotransplantation of the kidney from 33 to 671 days after PTRA, with a mean of 203 days.

2.5.1
Percutaneous Transluminal Renal Angioplasty of the In Situ Kidney

Patients previously treated with unilateral autotransplantation for renal artery stenosis are at increased risk of new stenosis in the contralateral (in situ) kidney. Such

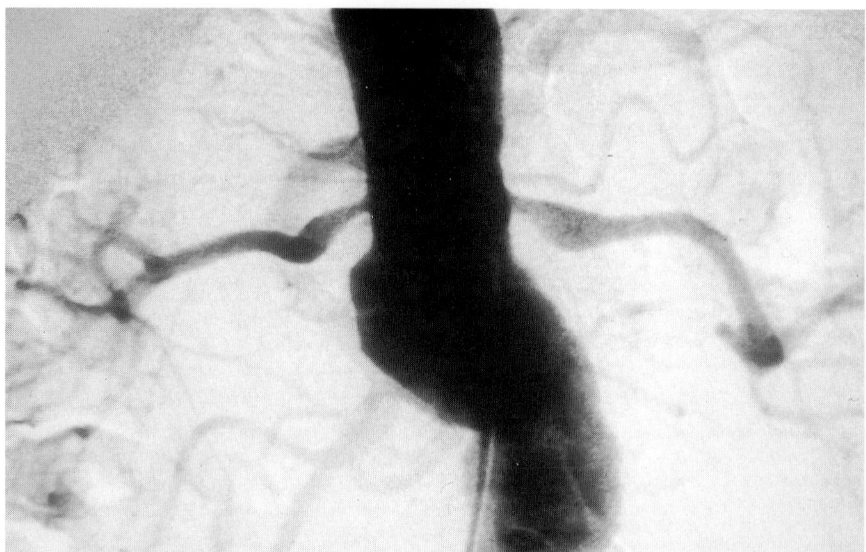

Fig. 2.13. Patient with an aortic aneurysm and bilateral renal artery stenosis. Bilateral balloon angioplasty in this patient resulted in multiple infarctions of the right kidney and restenosis bilaterally. Four months later the patient was successfully treated with aortoiliac bypass and renal autotransplantation

lesions should be suspected whenever worsening or recurrence of the hypertension is diagnosed. The indication for treatment, and the PTRA technique to be used do not differ from that for a previously untreated patient (Fig. 2.14). We have treated eight patients for stenosis in the remaining in situ kidney. Six patients were successfully treated by one PTRA, and one patient after three PTRAs. In one patient the attempt was unsuccessful. The PTRAs were performed 1.72 ± 1.85 years after autotransplantation (range 57 days to 5.05 years).

2.5.2
Percutaneous Transluminal Renal Angioplasty of the Autotransplanted Kidney

New stenoses may evolve in the iliac artery, in the anastomosis between the renal and the iliac artery, and in the renal artery. PTRA can be performed successfully in most of these stenoses (Fig. 2.15). From 1982, we have treated 14 patients for arterial stenosis in a renal autotransplant (Table 2.1). The stenosis was located in the iliac artery in three patients, at or near the anastomosis in six, and in the renal artery in seven. In one patient, both the iliac artery and the anastomosis area were dilated, and in another, both the anastomosis area and the renal artery distal to the anastomosis were treated. The PTRA was successful in 13 patients and unsuccessful in one, who had stenosis in a segmental branch of the renal artery. PTRA was performed 65 days to 10.9 years, (mean 3.1 years) after autotransplantation. Only four patients were treated within 6 months after transplantation (65, 105, 113, and 126 days thereafter, respectively). No complications were seen in these patients. During the same period we performed 76 PTRAs for renal allotransplant arterial stenosis in 59 patients (Fauchald et al. 1992).

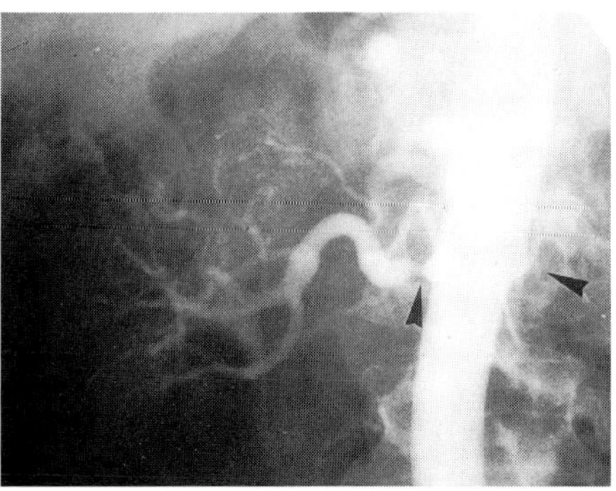
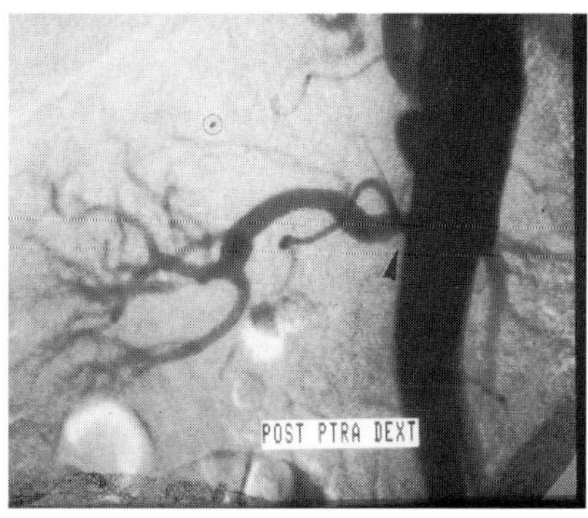

A   B

Fig. 2.14A,B. Balloon angioplasty of a stenosis in the right renal artery (→), before (A) and after (B) balloon dilatation. The patient had previously been successfully treated with autotransplantation of the left kidney for renal artery stenosis. Note the occluded left renal artery (→)

PTRAs of the internal iliac and renal arteries of transplanted kidneys are usually performed using a crossover technique, i.e., the femoral artery is punctured on the contralateral side to the transplanted kidney (Fig. 2.16). Ipsilateral puncture complicates selective catheterization because of the sharp angle between the external and the internal iliac arteries or between the external iliac and the renal artery. We always use a guide catheter technique to pass tight stenoses. Furthermore, this permits the use of a double guide wire technique to protect branches of the renal artery. The guide catheter is usually directed across the abdominal aortic bifurcation into the first part of internal iliac artery. Ipsilateral puncture is suitable for stenoses in the common iliac artery.

Early postoperative arterial stenosis usually occurs at the site of the anastomosis as a result of the surgical technique or the formation of an intimal crest. While these stenoses are easily treated by PTRA, arterial kinking is difficult to treat with balloons

Table 2.1. Percutaneous transluminal renal angioplasty (PTRA) in autotransplanted kidneys

Number of PTRAs	21
Total patients	14
Men (%)	5 (36)
Women (%)	9 (64)
Mean age years (range)	48 (24-69)
Arterial segments treated	16
Internal iliac artery	3
Anastomosis region	6
Renal artery	7
Time from autotransplantation to PTRA	
Mean years (range)	3.1 (65 days-11 years)
0-6 months (no. of patients)	4
6-12 months (no. of patients)	2
1-5 years (no. of patients)	4
>5 years (no. of patients)	4
Results	
Primary technical success rate	20/21 (95%)
Successfully treated patients (final result after the last PTRA)	13/14 (93%)

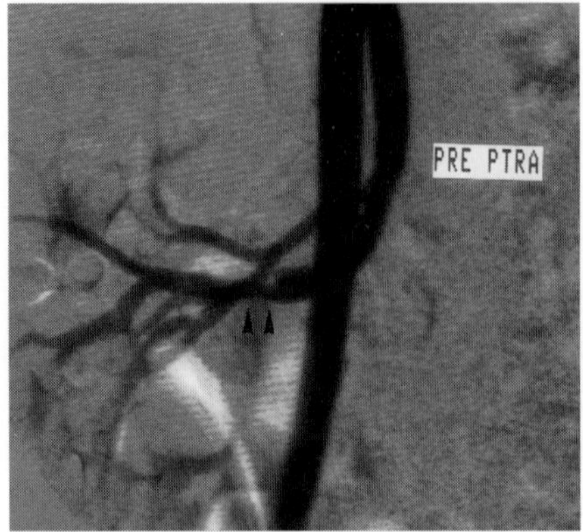

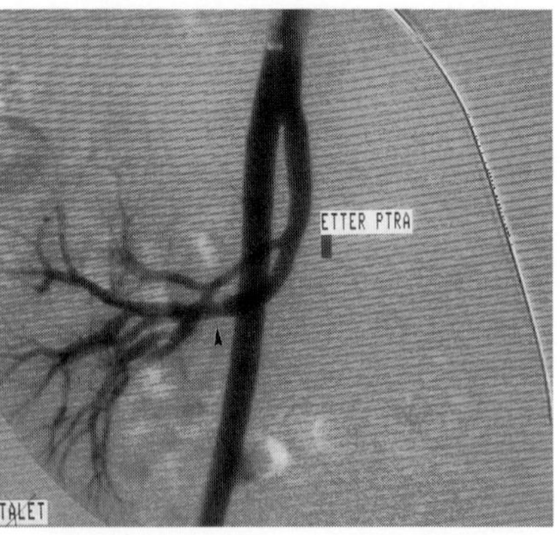

Fig. 2.15A,B. Balloon angioplasty of a stenosis (→) in a renal transplant artery anastomosed to the right internal iliac artery, before (A) and after (B) dilatation. The guide catheter has been advanced from the left femoral artery, over the aortic bifurcation, and positioned in the right common iliac artery

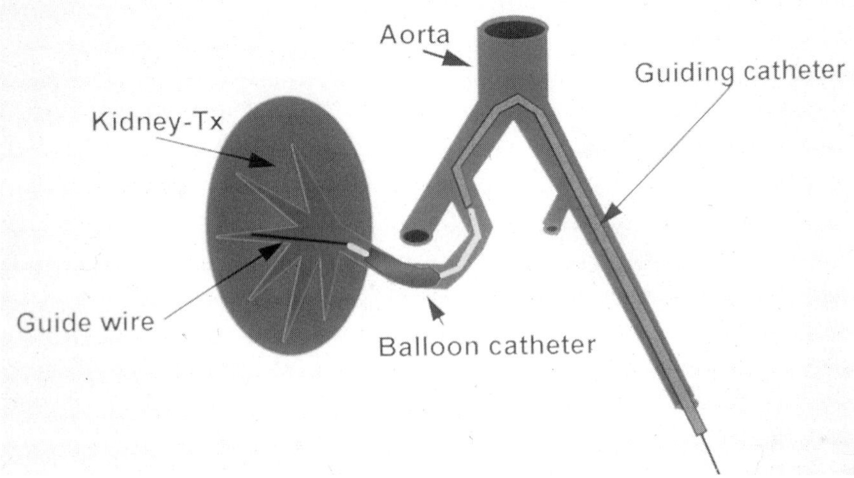

Fig. 2.16. Percutaneous transluminal angioplasty of a renal transplant artery using guide catheter assisted angioplasty and cross-over technique. The femoral artery has been punctured at the contralateral side and the guide catheter is positioned in the ostium of the right internal iliac artery (from Kløw and Vatne 1994)

alone because the kinking usually recoils. In these cases, intravascular stents may be used. Sometimes it is difficult from the angiographic appearance to discriminate between stenosis and kinking. Characteristically, the balloon is easily expanded during balloon inflation in a kinked artery. After deflation, however, the kinking recoils and the angiographic appearance is usually unchanged.

2.6
Conclusions

Hypertension and deterioration of renal function caused by renal artery abnormalities can be treated successfully by PTRA or renal autotransplantation and should thus be diagnosed at the earliest possible stage. PTRA is now the primary and definitive treatment for the majority of renal artery lesions. Surgical correction of the arterial lesion is indicated in cases unsuitable for PTRA or when PTRA has failed.

Several noninvasive tests may be used to identify patients with renal artery abnormalities. Presently, however, only intraarterial renal angiography gives reliable and sufficiently detailed information needed for surgery or angioplasty. For postoperative investigations, several methods may be used such as sonography, urography, CT, duplex sonography, MR angiography, and CT angiography, to check for arterial or venous patency, adequate drainage of urine, possible urine leakage, and hematoma or lymphocele formation.

References

Barrett BJ, Carlisle EJ (1993) Metaanalysis of the relative nephrotoxicity of high- and low-osmolality iodinated contrast media. Radiology 188:171-178

Bluemke DA, Chambers TP (1995) Spiral CT angiography: an alternative to conventional angiography. Radiology 195:317-319

Brekke IB, Sødal G, Jakobsen A, et al. (1992) Fibro-muscular renal artery disease treated by extracorporeal vascular reconstruction and renal autotransplantation: short- and long-term results. Eur J Vasc Surg 6:471-476

Debatin JF, Spritzer CE, Grist TM, et al. (1991) Imaging of the renal arteries: value of MR angiography. AJR 157:981-990

Dorros G, Prince C, Mathiak L (1993) Stenting of a renal artery stenosis achieves better relief of the obstructive lesion than balloon angioplasty. Cathet Cardiovasc Diagn 29:191-198

Tauchald P, Vatne K, Paulsen D, et al. (1992) Long-term clinical results of percutaneous transluminal angioplasty in transplant renal artery stenosis. Nephrol Dial Transplant 7:256-259

Flatmark A, Albrechtsen D, Sødal G et al. (1989) Renal autotransplantation. World J Surg 13:206-210

Frauchiger B, Bock A, Spoendlin M, et al. (1994) Early renal transplant dysfunction due to arterial kinking stenosis. Nephrol Dial Transplant 9:76-79

Grüntzig AR, Kuhlman U, Vetter W, et al. (1978) Treatment of renovascular hypertension with percutaneous transluminal dilatation of a renal artery stenosis. Lancet 1:801-802

Havey RJ, Krumlosky F, del Graco F, et al. (1985) Screening for renovascular hypertension. Is renal digital-subtraction angiography the preferred noninvasive test? JAMA 254:388-393

Jensen G, Zachrisson BF, Delin K, et al (1995) Treatment of renovascular hypertension: one year results of renal angioplasty. Kidney Int 48:1936-1945

Katzen BT (1995) Current status of digital angiography in vascular imaging. Radiol Clin North Am 33:1-14

Kjellevand TO, Kolmannskog F, Pfeffer P, et al. (1991) Influence of renal angiography in living potential kidney donors. Acta Radiol 32:368-370

Kliewer MA, Tupler RH, Carroll BA, et al. (1993) Renal artery stenosis: analysis of Doppler waveform parameters and tardus-parvus pattern. Radiology 189:779-787

Kløw NE, Levorstad K, Berg KJ, et al. (1993) Iodixanol in cardioangiography in patients with coronary artery disease: tolerability, cardiac and renal effects. Acta Radiol 34:72-77

Kløw NE, Vatne K (1994) Stenoses of the renal arteries treated with catheters. Tidsskr Nor Lægeforen 114:2728-2731

Korogi Y, Takahashi M (1993) A double-guide-wire technique in renal angioplasty. Acta Radiol 34:196-197

Krestin GP (1994) Magnetic resonance imaging of the kidneys: current status. Magn Reson Q 10:2-21

Novick AC, Ziegelbaum M, Vidt DG, et al. (1987) Trends in surgical revascularization for renal artery disease: ten years experience. JAMA 257:498-501

Palmaz JC, Kopp DT, Hayashi H, et al. (1987) Normal and stenotic renal arteries: experimental balloon-expandable intraluminal stenting. Radiology 164:705-708

Pickering TG (1991) Diagnosis and evaluation of renovascular hypertension: indication for therapy. Circulation 83[Suppl I]:I147-154

Rubin GD, Dake MD, Semba CP (1995) Current status of three-dimensional spiral CT scanning for imaging the vasculature. Radiol Clin North Am 33:51-70

Saarinen O, Salmela K, Edgren J (1994) Doppler ultrasound in the diagnosis of renal transplant artery stenosis - value of resistive index. Acta Radiol 35:586-589

Schmitz-Rode T, Günther RW, Keulers P (1993) Angiographie und Druckmessung bei koaxialem Gleitführungsdraht: Kontrolle nach Nierenangioplastie. Fortschr Röntgenstr 158:74-75

Schwerk WB, Restrepo IK, Stellwaag M, et al. (1994) Renal artery stenosis: grading with image-directed Doppler US. Evaluation of renal resistive index. Radiology 190: 780-790

Smith HJ, Bakke SJ (1993) MR angiography of in situ and transplanted renal arteries. Acta Radiol 34:150-155

Snider JF, Hunter DW, Moradian GP, et al. (1989) Transplant renal artery stenosis: evaluation with duplex sonography. Radiology 172:1027-1030

Soulen MC (1994) Renal angioplasty: underutilized or overvalued? Radiology 193: 19-21

Tegtmeyer CJ, Selby JB, Hartwell GD et al. (1991) Results and complications of angioplasty in fibromuscular dysplasia. Circulation 83[Suppl I]:I155-161

Tollefson DFJ, Ernst CB (1991) Natural history of atherosclerotic artery stenosis associated with aortic disease. J Vasc Surg 14:327-331

Weibull H, Bergqvist D, Bergentz SE, et al. (1993) Percutaneous transluminal angioplasty versus surgical reconstruction of atherosclerotic renal artery stenosis: a prospective randomized study. J Vasc Surg 18:841-852

White CJ, Ramee SR, Collins TJ, et al. (1991) Guide catheter-assisted renal artery angioplasty. Cathet Cardiovasc Diagn 23:10-13

Renal Radionuclide Studies

Jan G. Fjeld and Kjell Rootwelt

3.1
Introduction

Radionuclide methods are important diagnostic modalities for the detection and quantification of renal disease. There are three categories of renal radionuclide investigations:

- Clearance studies
- Split function investigations with measurement of parenchymal uptake, parenchymal wash-out, and pelvic and ureteric urinary flow (renography)
- Renal imaging (scintigraphy)

All the diagnostic modalities offered by a department of nuclear medicine can be performed on an out-patient basis. The methods give results that help the physician to choose between surgical or conservative management of renal disease. Moreover, if surgery is the choice, these methods may assist the surgeon in deciding whether autotransplantation should be considered. The indications for preoperative studies thus include all the diseases that may lead to renal autotransplantation, and the preoperative work up includes methods from all three categories above.

Postoperatively, renal radionuclide methods are used to examine the function of the kidney transplant in its new location immediately after the operation, and to monitor transplant function during long-term follow-up.

3.1.1
Radiopharmaceuticals

Technetium-99m is the radionuclide of choice in nuclear medicine. With its 140 keV gamma energy, this radioisotope has optimum energy for the gamma camera. Technetium is also preferred because of its availability; a technetium-99m generator is obligatory in every department of nuclear medicine. The technetium-99m generator provides the department with daily eluates of technetium-99m in the form of sodium pertechnetate, which is used as a labeling agent for a large number of pharmaceuticals. The presently available renal agents for technetium labeling are diethylene-triamine-penta-acetate (DTPA) for determination of glomerular filtration rate (GFR), mercaptoacetyltriglycine (MAG3) for renography, and dimercapto-succinic acid (DMSA) for static parenchymal imaging.

Technetium-99m-MAG3 has a high protein binding in plasma, a low volume of distribution, and is mainly excreted in the urine by tubular secretion and only to a minor degree by glomerular filtration (Rehling et al. 1995). The agent gives a high kidney to background ratio, providing better images of the kidneys and urinary system than technetium-99m-DTPA. It is thus excellent for determination of split kidney function when both kidneys are in situ.

Only 15% of the technetium-99m-DMSA is excreted by ultrafiltration, and this ultrafiltrated fraction is not reabsorbed. There is no tubular secretion. On the other hand, the tubular cells extract and retain technetium-99m-DMSA from the peritubular fluid (Müller-Suur and Gutsche 1995). Normally, approximately 40% of the injected dose is retained (Groshar et al. 1989). The decrease in kidney activity after 2-3 h can be almost completely accounted for by physical decay. Technetium-99m-DMSA has become the agent of choice for high-quality static imaging of the renal cortex and estimation of functioning renal mass.

None of the technetium-99m-labeled renal agents are extracted quantitatively in the kidneys, and if a measurement of effective renal plasma flow (ERPF) is needed, radioactive ortho-iodo-hippurate (OIH) should be used. Either I-131 or I-123 can be used as the label.

3.1.2
Equipment

3.1.2.1
Probe Detectors

Probe detectors are simple scintillation detectors used for registering the count rate over a limited field of view. Their use in renal studies is limited to clearance estimations performed by continuous external recording of the decrease in count rate from extrarenal tissue.

3.1.2.2
Well Scintillation Counters

Plasma samples are counted in well scintillation counters. These are either of a multiwell or an automatic sample changer type.

3.1.2.3
Gamma Cameras

Gamma cameras are the workhorses of every department of nuclear medicine. They are used for planar scintigraphy and for single photon emission computer tomography (SPECT). The gamma cameras are also used for dynamic studies (i.e., renographies), where the results are presented as multiple serial scintigrams acquired during the observation period and as time-activity curves (renograms). The serial images give morphological information that helps to distinguish between prerenal, parenchymatous, and obstructive disorders.

3.2
Basic Principles for Quantitative Evaluation

3.2.1
Blood Sampling Methods

The plasma clearance of radiopharmaceuticals can be determined by counting blood samples collected at intervals after a bolus intravenous injection. Provided the radiopharmaceutical is excreted only through the kidneys, renal clearance can be calculated by dividing the injected activity by the area under the plasma time-activity curve.

When an exact measurement of GFR and ERPF is needed, biexponential analysis of the plasma time-activity curve is recommended (Sapirstein et al. 1955). The radiopharmaceuticals technetium-99m-DTPA and I-131-OIH may be injected at the same time, allowing simultaneous determination of GFR and ERPF. The filtration fraction may be calculated from these two parameters.

Biexponential analysis requires multiple plasma samples - occasionally collected for up to 24 h - and is inconvenient in a busy clinical routine. Simplified methods based on a single compartment model and one or two plasma samples have therefore been introduced. The initial plasma concentration (i.e., the count rate at time zero) can be predicted from the injected dose and the body dimensions, as described by Bubeck et al. (1992). Then only a single blood sample is needed to estimate the plasma clearance. One might, nevertheless, prefer to withdraw two blood samples and obtain the monoexponential slope directly or to calculate two parallel estimates of the clearance.

3.2.2
Extrarenal Surface Activity Measurement

Extrarenal surface counting may be used to estimate kidney function as an alternative (or supplement) to plasma sampling. A convenient way is to place a single anterior probe over the upper part of the thorax, recording the radioactivity disappearance rate in the central thoracic blood vessels. The decrease in activity from 10 to 20 min after the radiopharmaceutical injection can be used to estimate ERPF when either I-131-OIH or technetium-99m-MAG3 is used as the radiopharmaceutical. The activity decreases monoexponentially between 10 and 20 min, and the exponential constant of the equation describing this decrease, multiplied by 10^4, is numerically close to ERPF/1.73 m^2 body surface. A more exact value can be read from an empiric nomogram. The thorax activity curve is convenient to use as an independent check on the plasma sampling method.

3.2.3
Kidney Uptake

Vendors of gamma camera software deliver programs that allow the user to estimate total kidney function from the initial kidney uptake. The syringe with the patient's dose is counted with the gamma camera before the i.v. injection. Thereafter, acquisition is performed dynamically with the gamma camera over the kidneys. Kidney activity is recorded from regions of interest (ROIs) drawn around each kidney, and time-activity curves are constructed. The activity curves have to be corrected for the circulating background activity. The absolute as well as relative function of each kidney can be estimated from the initial phase of the net kidney curves. For absolute function calculations, the net kidney uptakes have to be corrected for attenuation. Kidney depth is estimated from the patient weight and height. When technetium-99m-DTPA is used, the calculations are based on the method described by Gates (1982), and the Schlegel method (1979) is used with I-131-OIH. We have found that when using technetium-99m-MAG3 on kidneys in situ, the Schlegel algorithms may be used without modification. The numerical results will be equal to the ERPF and not to the technetium-99m-MAG3 clearance (Rootwelt 1990). Since kidneys transplanted to the iliac fossa are closer to the body surface, tissue attenuation will be lower and the apparent net kidney uptake and ERPF erroneously high. We multiply the ERPF by a factor of 0.6 to correct for this. This simplification is reasonably accurate to an acceptable degree of precision.

A patient treated with renal autotransplantation may or may not have the contralateral kidney in situ. In a few cases both kidneys are autotransplanted. The relative function of a transplant in the iliac fossa and a kidney in situ, or of two transplants, can also be estimated. However, the different locations of the transplant and in situ kidney have a significant impact on the relative count rate, as recorded with an external probe detector or gamma camera. The difference in depth from skin to kidney gives a difference in tissue attenuation. This can be corrected for by calculating the geometrical mean of anterior and posterior count rates for each kidney (Taylor 1982; Wuzanto et al. 1987). However, with the radiopharmaceuticals technetium-99m-MAG3 and technetium-99m-DTPA, there is a dynamic situation with rapid changes in the renal input and output rates. Consequently, count rates recorded with the camera in both the dorsal and ventral positions are not comparable, because the measurements are made during different time intervals. This is coped with by using technetium-99m-DMSA, which gives a relatively static parenchymatous content in the period 3-24 h after the injection.

3.2.4
Transit Times

Numerical analysis is used to characterize the pattern of the net renographic time-activity curve and for objective comparison between studies performed successively. Two useful and simple parameters are the time from injection to peak activity and the T1/2 for the subsequent activity fall. More refined indices may also be extracted. However, the time to peak activity and T1/2 usually suffice, provided visual evaluation of sequential images is included. When there is a delay in the start of excretion of radioactivity, parenchymal retention may then be differentiated from dilated or obstructed uropathy.

3.3
Clinical Procedures: Methodology

3.3.1
Glomerular Filtration Rate (GFR)

The patient should neither eat nor smoke during the preceding 4 h. Fluids, with the exception of tea or coffee, are allowed. The procedure is started with a bolus i.v. injection of 40 MBq technetium-99m-DTPA, followed by six blood samples taken from the recumbent patient 5, 15, 120, 150, 180 and 210 min after the injection. In patients with ascites, edema, or markedly reduced kidney function (serum creatinine > 300 µmol/l), blood samples are also taken after 6 and 24 h. GFR is calculated by the method of Sapirstein et al. (1955) and compared to age-adjusted reference ranges.

The method's coefficient of variation is approximately 10% in the GFR range 30–90 ml/min per 1.73 m2 body surface. The effective dose is 0.2 mSv.

3.3.2
Renography

Renography is the standard method for estimation of split renal function. No restriction in food or fluid intake is necessary prior to the investigation. The i.v. injection of technetium-99m-MAG3 is 3 MBq/kg body weight (maximum 100 MBq). The patient lies supine, and dynamic acquisition is performed for 24 min with the gamma camera detector dorsally. Simultaneous extrarenal activity disappearance is recorded with a single probe detector located over the thorax. Blood samples are drawn at 25 and 35 min. Total kidney function is estimated (Bubeck et al. 1992) and compared with function estimates derived from the thorax activity curve and the net kidney uptake measurement during the period 1-2 min after the injection. Split kidney function is calculated from the same net kidney uptake values. Net time activity curves are processed with measurement of time to peak activity and T1/2. Serial scintiphotos are evaluated for space occupying lesions, infarction, scars, etc., as well as for hydronephrosis or other kinds of pathology in the upper urinary tract.

The technetium-99m-MAG3 clearance is in essence an estimate of the tubular excretory capacity. The clearance generally varies in proportion to ERPF (correlation coefficient 0.95-0.98) and GFR, giving values that are approximately 55% and 275% of ERPF and GFR, respectively. Total renal function estimates should not be lower than 30% below the age-adjusted reference mean, and asymmetry in kidney function should not exceed 44%/56%. Time to peak activity should be below 6 min, and T1/2 below 15 min. Total function estimates are inaccurate when kidney function is worse than 10% of the reference mean. When total function is better, follow-up changes exceeding 10% of the reference mean are considered significant. Single kidney relative function must change 6 percentage points to be considered significant. The effective dose is 0.7 mSv/100 MBq.

3.3.3
Intervention Renographies

3.3.3.1
Diuresis Renography

Diuresis renography is a modification of ordinary renography chosen when urinary tract abnormalities are suspected. The rationale behind the diuresis augmentation is given in Sect. 3.4.2. The patient should drink 20 ml/kg body weight during the 60 min period preceding the injection of technetium-99m-MAG3. Furthermore, furosemid (1 mg/kg body weight up to 20 kg; 20 mg for body weight 20-40 kg; 0.5 mg/kg for body weight over 40 kg, but not exceeding 40 mg) is injected i.v. 10 min after the technetium-99m-MAG3. The bladder should be emptied before the technetium-99m-MAG3 injection. Diuretic response is measured by a second bladder emptying at the end of the gamma camera acquisition.

Net kidney activity should start to fall within 1-2 min after the furosemid injection. As a rule of thumb, the activity should thereafter fall exponentially with a $T_{1/2}$ of less than 10 min. Definite pathology is reflected as an increase in kidney activity or a slow decrease with a $T_{1/2}$ longer than 20 min. In approximately 15% of the studies, indeterminate gray zone values are found. The poorer the kidney function, the poorer is the discriminatory power of diuresis renography.

3.3.3.2
Captopril Renography

Captopril renography is a modification of ordinary renography chosen when renal artery stenosis is a possible or known diagnosis. The rationale behind captopril-augmented renography is discussed in Sect. 3.4.1. The patient should not eat during the preceding 4 h. An i.v. infusion of 0.9% saline is established as a precaution in case excessive captopril causes a fall in blood pressure. A 25 mg tablet of captopril is chewed and swallowed, followed by drinking 1 liter of water during the next 60 min. Blood pressure is measured every 15 min. After bladder emptying, technetium-99m-MAG3 is injected i.v.

The renal time-activity curves will usually change in kidneys supplied by renal arteries with a hemodynamicaly significant stenosis. The time to maximum activity increases more than 1 min, the $T_{1/2}$ becomes prolonged, and the serial scintiphotos usually show the affected kidney somewhat smaller than the contralateral kidney. The dynamic images may disclose branch stenoses even if the renal time-activity curve is not changed significantly. The method has a sensitivity of only 50%-70% for anatomical renal artery stenosis. However, when the stenosis exceeds 70%, the sensitivity is 90%, and the predictive value for an antihypertensive effect of successful revascularization is 93% (Fommei et al. 1991). Bilateral changes impose a diagnostic problem, and the specificity of 80%-85% is not too impressive. Specificity can be improved by using technetium-99m-DTPA and performing two sequential renographies, one with and the second without captopril.

3.3.4
Autotransplant Renography

Renographic investigation of a kidney autotransplanted to the iliac region can be performed like an ordinary renography, the only exception being that the gamma camera detector must be positioned ventrally to acquire the transplant count rate. Dynamic scintigrams and the time-activity curve should disclose anoxic damage, vascular obstruction, urinary leaks, lymphoceles, hematomas, or urinomas. However, determination of split renal function is not possible with this modified renography. For this purpose 75 MBq technetium-99m-DMSA is injected i.v. the previous afternoon. The next morning, static gamma camera recording is performed from both behind and in front of the autotransplant, as well as from the kidney in situ. The relative kidney function is calculated from the geometric means of the respective anterior and posterior count rates. Thereafter, technetium-99m-MAG3 renography is performed over the autotransplant. If both kidneys are autotransplanted, their depths are similar, and technetium-99m-DMSA injection is unnecessary. The effective dose of the combined study is 1.7 mSv.

3.4
Selected Procedures in the Preoperative Work-up

3.4.1
Renovascular Disease

When renovascular hypertension is suspected, captopril-augmented renography is preferred. A renal artery stenosis with functional consequences gives an abnormality in the renogram because the poststenotic hydrostatic pressure is decreased. This gives not only a lower filtration pressure over the glomerular membrane, but also a decrease in the peritubular pressure, increasing the reabsorption of water and salts. Hence, the mean transit time of radiopharmaceuticals tends to be longer in a kidney with renovascular disease than in normal kidneys. A 1-min delay in the transit time, relative to the other kidney, may be a significant sign of stenosis. Figure 3.1 illustrates the renographic findings in a patient with unilateral renovascular disease.

With more moderate renovascular pathology, the renographic findings are often less evident than in Fig. 3.1. The reason for this is that renal autoregulatory mechanisms are activated to restore the filtration pressure, leading to contraction of the efferent arterioles from the glomerulus. The regulatory mechanism behind this is the following cascade of reactions: when the filtration pressure is diminished, the juxtaglomerular apparatus produces and releases renin, which cleaves angiotensinogen to angiotensin I, which, in turn, is converted by angiotensin converting enzyme (ACE) in the lungs into the vasoconstrictor angiotensin II. This renal autoregulation affects the renogram, making the renographic characteristics less evident. However, if ACE-inhibitory medication is administered, the efferent arterioles are dilated and the filtration pressure is decreased. Therefore, when the stenosis is one-sided, ACE inhibitors exaggerate the differences in the renograms of the two kidneys. Hence, ACE inhibitors increase the sensitivity of renography. Three ACE inhibitors are on the market

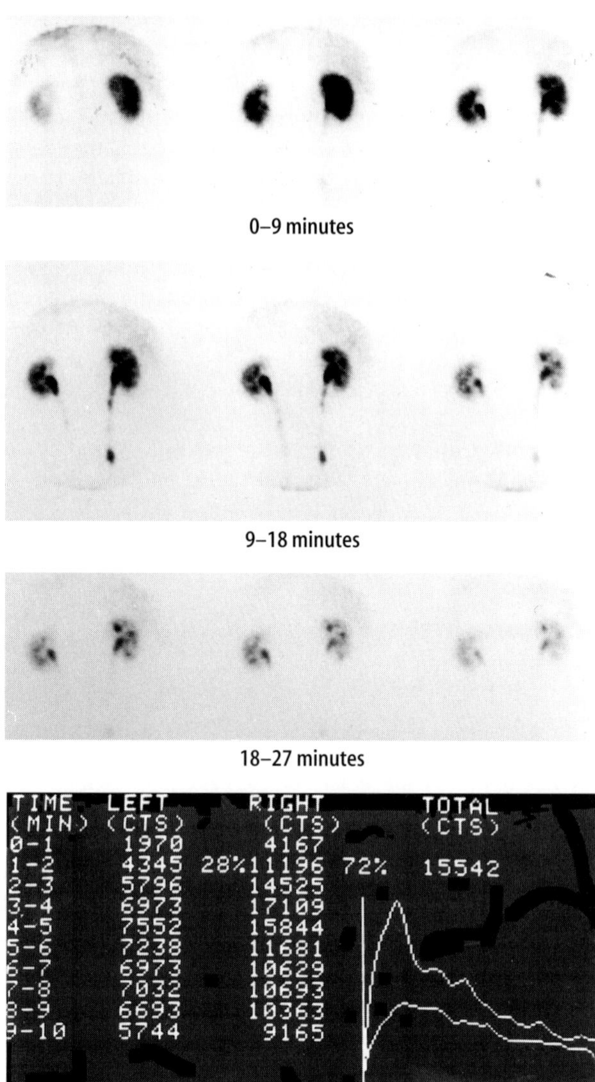

Fig. 3.1. Serial scintiphotos (kidneys and bladder, dorsal view) and time-activity curves (renograms) from technetium-99m-MAG3 renography (without captopril) in a 42-year-old hypertensive man with renal artery stenosis. Renal angiography had shown subtotal stenosis of the left renal artery. Percutaneous transluminal renal angioplasty (PTRA) with stent implantation was performed 5 days before renography. Nevertheless, the left kidney, relative to the right, shows a marked reduction in uptake, delay in time to peak activity (3 vs. 4 min), and prolonged half-time during washout (8 vs. 15 min). Split function left/right kidney was estimated at 28%/72%.

One year after this renography, it was decided to autotransplant the left kidney to the left iliac fossa. Three months after the operation, autotransplant renography showed that the split function between the autotransplant and the kidney in situ was 41%/59%, and the autotransplant renography gave a time to peak activity of 3 min, and a washout half-time of 13 min today: captopril, enalapril, and lisinopril. The effect is faster and has a shorter duration with captopril than with the other two, and captopril is therefore preferred for these studies. Since technetium-99m-DTPA is a purely glomerular-filtered agent, the post-captopril renography demonstrates a marked reduction in uptake on the affected side, as well as a delay in the time to peak activity, and a prolongation of T1/2. A tubular agent such as technetium-99m-MAG3 mainly demonstrates progressive accumulation and delayed excretion in the post-captopril study, but not a very marked decrease in kidney uptake. Total renal function should be determined as GFR (Sect. 3.3.1) .

3.4.2
Urinary Obstruction

Diuretic-augmented renography is used primarily for the diagnosis of pelvi-ureteric junction stenosis or any other cause of ureteric obstruction, and it is particularly useful for the evaluation of the effect of urological surgery on the upper urinary tract flow. When the urinary pathway is dilated, ordinary renography is poorly suited to differentiate between an obstructed and a nonobstructed system. The time to peak activity and the T1/2 may be increased to the same extent. However, the i.v. administration of diuretics (furosemid) will normally increase diuresis to 7-10 ml/min or more, which will lead to a rapid washout of activity from a nonobstructed (Fig. 3.2), but not from an obstructed system (Fig. 3.3). Kidneys with urinary outflow obstruction are at risk, and a number of measures are usually needed to prevent the kidney function from deteriorating. Once again, GFR (Sect. 3.3.1) gives a more accurate estimate of the total kidney function than technetium-99m-MAG3 renography.

3.4.3
Renal Cancer

The advantage of the radionuclide methods is their functional information. A renal tumor may sometimes be detected as a space-occupying lesion on the scintiphotos, or it may be indirectly detected because it affects renal function. However, with respect to structural changes in the kidneys and the detection of tumors, the radionuclide methods are inferior to radiological methods, magnetic resonance, or ultrasound.

3.5
Autotransplant Follow-up

3.5.1
Total Renal Function

Just as in any other patient with a renal problem referred to the nuclear medicine department, ERPF and GFR are the most reliable radionuclide parameters for total renal function in an autotransplanted patient. The procedures are described above (Sect. 3.2.1). If the preoperative values of the same parameters are available, this helps to evaluate the effect of autotransplanation.

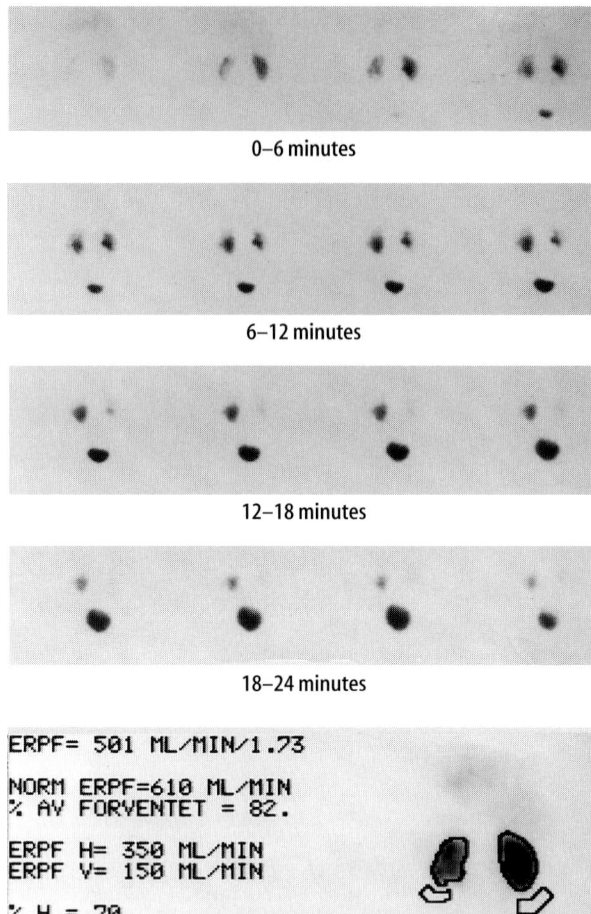

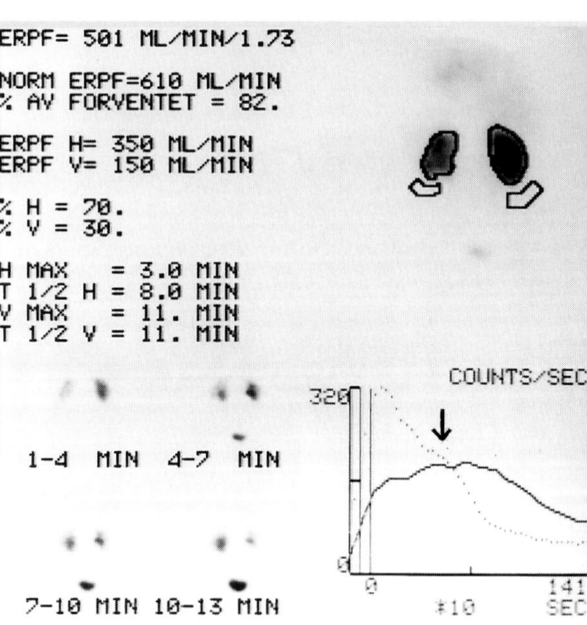

Fig. 3.2. Diuresis renography in a patient with hydronephrosis in the left kidney and a nonobstructed outflow system. Administration of furosemid after 10 min (arrow) induces increased washout. Normal kidney and outflow system on the right side

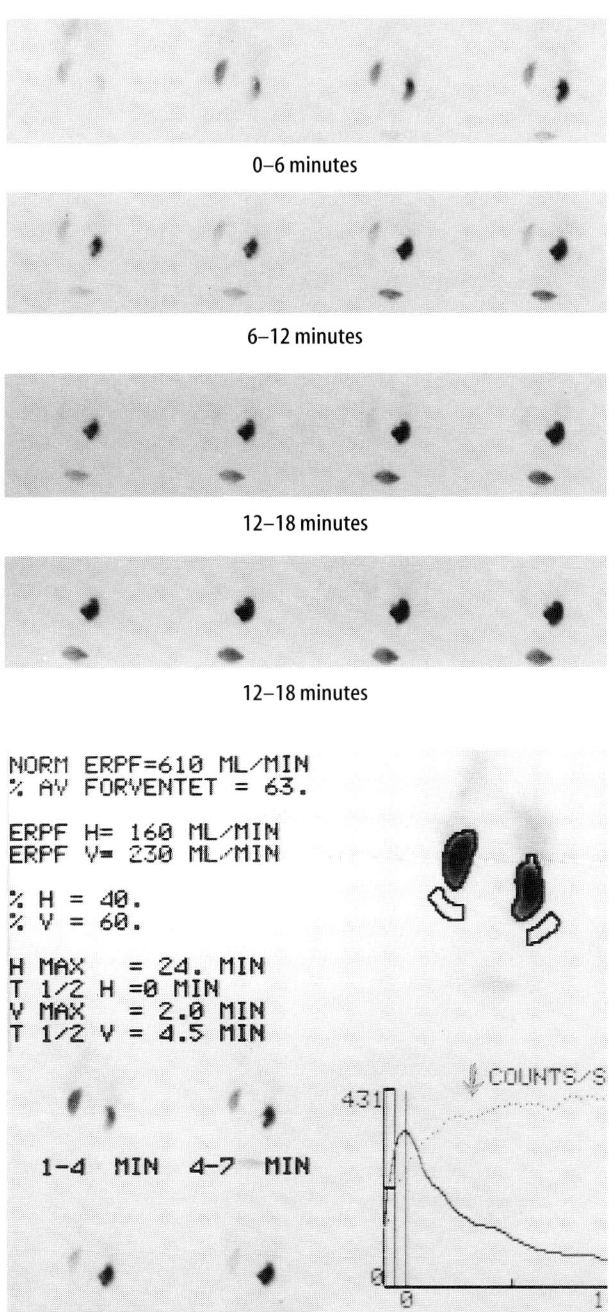

Fig. 3.3. Diuresis renography in a patient with hydronephrosis and obstruction on the right side: administration of furosemid (arrow) 10 min after the technetium-99m-MAG3 has no effect on the washout. Normal results on the left side

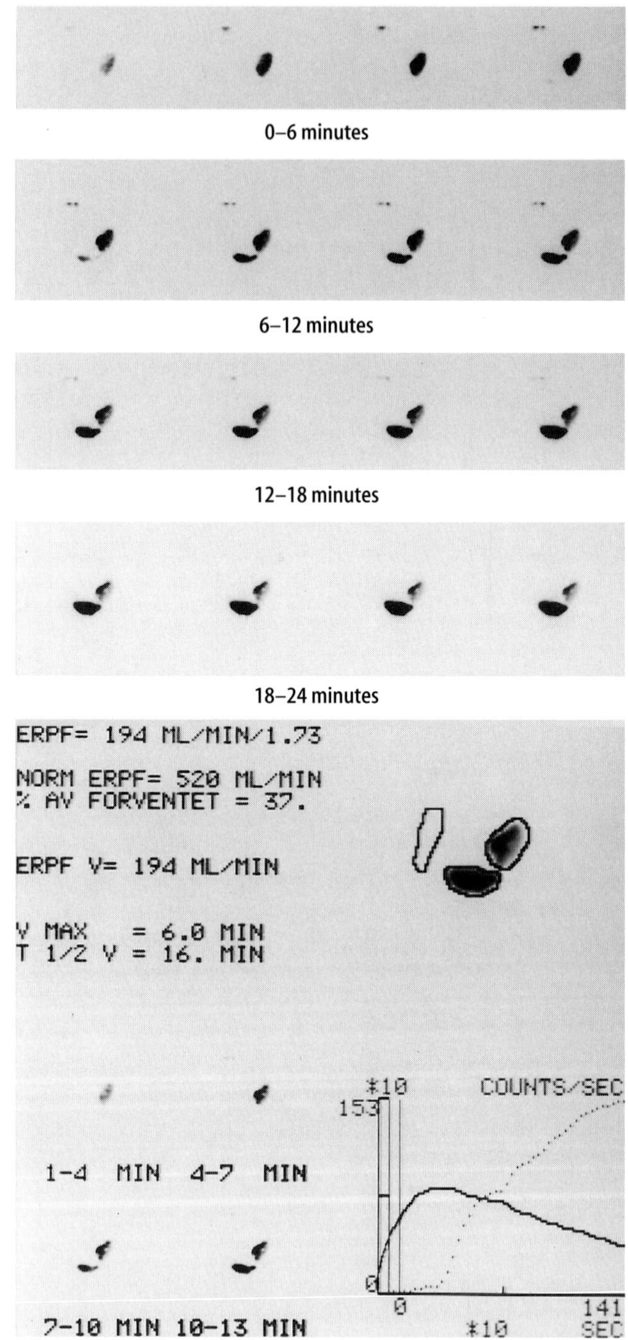

Fig. 3.4. Autotransplant renography in a 47-year-old woman with the left kidney transplanted to the left iliac fossa 5 years ago. Serial scintiphotos of transplant and bladder (ventral view), and renogram over the autotransplant. Dotted line represents the bladder activity

3.5.2
Autotransplant Function

The net autotransplant uptake values during the initial 1- to 2-min period give a gamma camera estimate of the autotransplant function (Sect. 3.2.3, Fig. 3.4).

A patient treated with renal autotransplantation may or may not have the contralateral kidney in situ. The split function of an autotransplant and a kidney in situ can be estimated if the difference in depth is corrected for by the use of geometrical mean values (Sect. 3.3.4). The patient in Fig. 3.4 has the right kidney in situ, and the split function of right kidney/autotransplant was 67%/33%. Knowing the relative function of the transplant, the GFR and ERPF of the transplant are obtained from the results of the blood-sampling methods (Sect. 3.2.1).

References

Bubeck B, Piepenburg R, Grethe U, Ehrig B, Hahn K (1992) A new principle to normalize plasma concentrations allowing single-sample-clearance determinations in both children and adults. Eur J Nucl Med 19:511-516

Fommei E, Mezzasalama L, Ghione S, Volterrani D, Oei Y, Hilson AJW, Carrieri M (1991) European captopril radionuclide test multicenter study. Preliminary results. Inspective renographic analysis. Am J Hypertens :S690-S697

Gates GF (1982) Glomerular filtration rate: estimation from fractional renal accumulation of 99mTc-DTPA (stannous). AJR 138:565-570

Groshar D, Frankel A, Iosilevsky G, Israel O, Moshovitz B, Levin DR, Front D (1989) Quanitation of renal uptake of technetium-99m-DMSA using SPECT. J Nucl Med 30:246-250

Müller-Suur R, Gutsche HU (1995) Tubular reabsorption of Technetium-99m-DMSA. J Nucl Med 36:1654-1658

Rehling M, Nielsen BU, Pedersen EB, Nielsen LE, Hansen HE, Bacher T (1995) Renal and extrarenal clearance of 99mTc-MAG3: a comparison with 125I-OIH and 51Cr-EDTA in patients representing all levels of glomerular filtration rate. Eur J Nucl Med 22:1379-1384

Rootwelt K (1990) Comparison of Tc-99m MAG3 and I-131 Hippuran for renal function studies. Eur J Nucl Med 16[Suppl];172

Sapirstein LA, Vidt DG, Mandel MJ, Hanusek G (1955) Volumes of distribution and clearances of intravenously injected creatinine in the dog. Am J Physiol 181:330-336

Schlegel JU, Halikiopoulos HL, Prima R (1979) Determination of filtration fraction using the gamma scintillation camera. J Urol 122:447-450

Taylor A (1982) Quantitation of renal function with static imaging agents. Semin Nucl Med 12:330-334

Wuzanto R, Lawson RS, Prescott M, et al. (1987) The importance of using anterior and posterior views in the calculation of differential renal function using 99mTc DMSA. Br J Radiol 60:869-872

Nephrectomy and Extracorporeal Renal Preservation: Technical Details

Bjørn Lien and Inge B. Brekke

4.1
Preoperative Evaluation and Preparation

Nephrectomy and extracorporeal renal surgery followed by renal autotransplantation must be considered a major surgical intervention. Therefore, a thorough preoperative evaluation of the patients general state of health is required with special emphasis on the cardiopulmonary status. Electrocardiography and chest X-ray should be performed in all patients over fifty. In patients with diabetes or atherosclerosis of the aorta or renal arteries, symptomatic or asymptomatic concomitant coronary heart disease should be excluded, as described in Chap. 10.

Treatment of any concomitant respiratory disease should be optimalized. This includes cessation of smoking as well as preoperative physiotherapy. A preoperative nonsmoking period of 2-3 weeks combined with physiotherapy and medical treatment should be recommended for patients with severe obstructive pulmonary disease. In this way, a significant improvement of the patient's respiratory condition can be achieved in most cases, thus reducing the risk of postoperative pulmonary complications.

4.2
Anatomical Considerations

The location of the superior renal pole is usually at the level of the twelfth thoracic vertebra, but may be as high as the tenth thoracic or as low as the second lumbar vertebra. The right kidney is usually situated 1-2 cm lower than the left. Together with the perinephric fat and the adrenal gland, each kidney is surrounded by a thin fascia (Gerota´s fascia). The cranial part of the kidneys are located above the inferior pleural deflection in close contact with the 11th and 12th ribs.

Variations in the renal vasculature are common (Olsson1986; Marshall 1986). In most cases a single renal artery arises from the aorta to supply each kidney, the right renal artery passing posterior to the inferior vena cava (IVC). The artery origin is usually slightly below, or at the level of the superior mesenteric artery (SMA). Before reaching the kidney, it gives off one or several branches supplying the adrenal gland, the perinephric tissue, the renal capsule and the ureter. Multiple renal arteries are encountered in approximately 30% of all individuals (Dyson 1995). They usually branch off the aorta between the SMA and the aortic bifurcation, but may in rare cases originate from the common iliac artery (Fig. 4.1). On the right side, accessory arteries may traverse ventral to the IVC. The various segments of the kidney are supplied by arteries that do not interconnect with neighboring segments, in contrast to the exten-

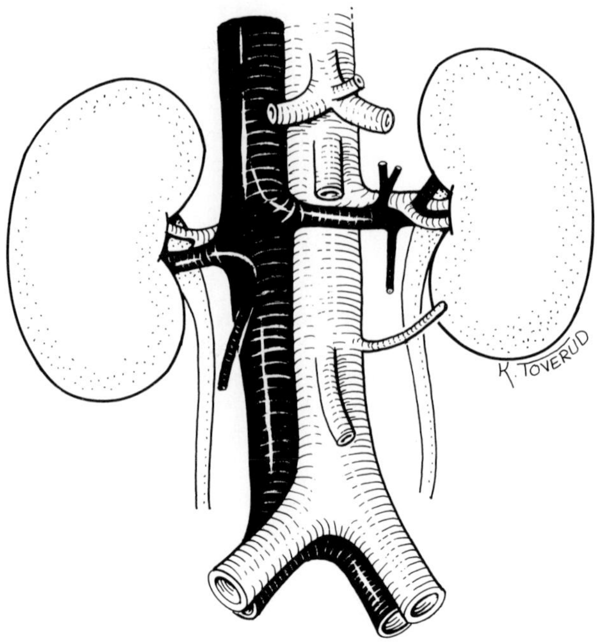

Fig. 4.1. Renal vascular supply. Accessory artery to the lower pole of the left kidney

sive intercommunication on the venous side. Occlusion of a renal artery will therefore inevitably be followed by ischemic necrosis of renal tissue. Consequently, all arteries of any significance must be preserved to avoid loss of renal parenchyma. Arteries supplying the inferior renal pole are of particular importance, as they usually represent the origin of the arterial supply to the ureter. Maximal length of all vessels must be obtained during nephrectomy to facilitate backtable vascular reconstruction. Gentle handling during dissection is of the utmost importance to avoid vascular spasm as well as disrupture of the vascular intimal lining.

The right renal vein is usually short, except in patients with a mobile kidney or unusually low renal placement. Multiple veins may be present, usually with separate drainage to the IVC. The left renal vein is longer than the right and rarely duplicated. It receives several tributaries: the gonadal vein, the adrenal vein, frequently one or more lumbar veins as well as several small veins from the perinephric tissue. A retro-aortic location of the left renal vein may occur. Two veins of equal size may be preserved, either on a common patch or by separate anastomoses. However, multiple collateral veins usually allow ligation of accessory veins without jeopardizing the renal circulation or inducing renal venous hypertension.

In horseshoe kidneys or kidneys with an anomalous location, the arterial supply may be bizarre (Perlmutter et al. 1986). A preoperative mapping by angiography is mandatory in all patients to be prepared for any abnormality of the vasculature. In rare cases, the inferior vena cava is duplicated (Fig. 4.2), the confluence being situated cranial to the renal veins. To avoid impaired venous return from the lower extremity as well as from the autotransplant, the left renal vein must in these cases be divided at an

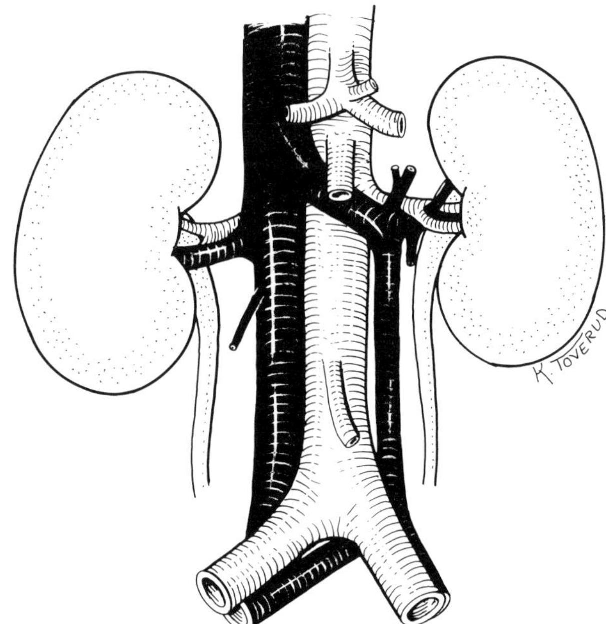

Fig. 4.2. Duplicated inferior vena cava

appropriate distance from the vena cava to allow closure of the central part of the vein without stenosis.

The ureters run from the renal pelvis inferiorly over the psoas muscle and cross the iliac vessels at the bifurcation of the internal and external iliac arteries. The main arterial supply comes from the renal arteries, but accessory vessels also come from the periureteral tissue and the gonadal vessels.

4.3
Nephrectomy: Technical Details

4.3.1
Choice of Incision

The nature of the renal disease to be treated, as well as its location, will determine the surgical approach and choice of incision. Previous renal or abdominal surgery, spinal deformity, or gross obesity may have an impact on this decision. Three different types of incisions, all common in renal surgery, may be used: the lateral (flank) (Fig. 4.3), the subcostal abdominal (transverse abdominal), or vertical midline incision (Fig. 4.4). All allow adequate exposure of the kidney, the renal vessels, and the ureter.

In unilateral nonmalignant renal disease, nephrectomy is performed through a flank incision. Bilateral disease is usually treated in a two-stage fashion. A three-month

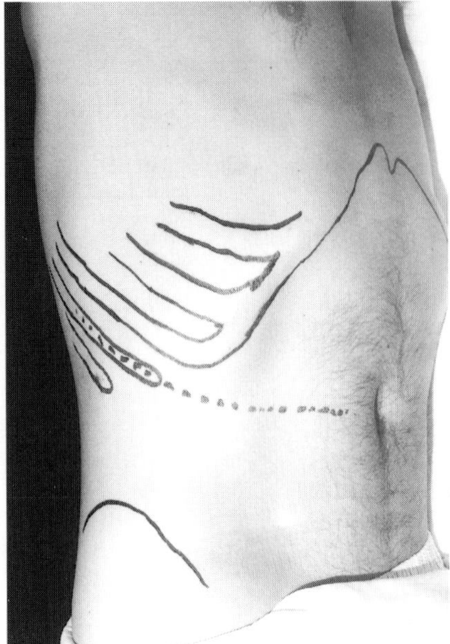

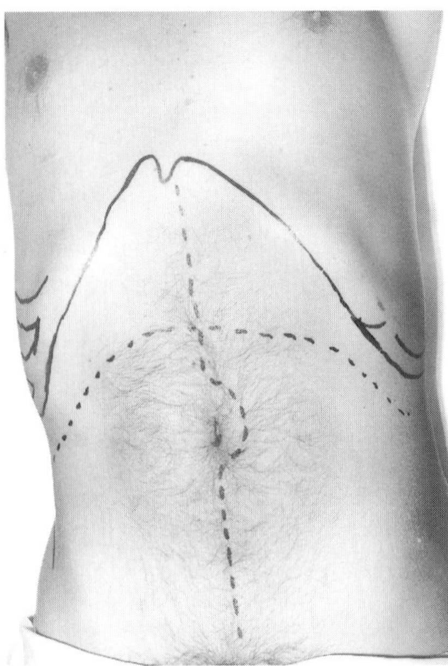

Fig. 4.3. The lateral (flank) incision (dotted line)

Fig. 4.4. Transverse abdominal and midline incisions (dotted lines)

interval between the autotransplantations allows full recovery of the patient and functional recovery of the autotransplant before the second operation. A flank incision is used in both operations.

When concomitant aortic surgery is required, a midline incision is preferred. If indicated, bilateral autotransplantation may then be performed as a one-stage procedure.

Nephrectomy in unilateral renal malignancy may be performed through a lateral incision, but large tumors are more easily removed using a subcostal or transverse abdominal incision. Patients presenting with bilateral tumors are best treated through a transverse abdominal rather than a midline incision.

4.3.1.1
Lateral (Flank) Incision

A retroperitoneal extrapleural approach with partial resection of the 11th rib is our standard incision in unilateral nephrectomy. Our experience with this incision in 1300 living-donor nephrectomies and 500 renal autotransplantations is that it allows adequate exposure of the kidney and the renal vessels. The wound healing is excellent and both early and late complications are rare.

With the patient in the flexed lateral decubitus position, the skin incision is made following the 11th rib from the mid-axillary line to the lateral border of the rectus abdominis muscle at the level of the umbilicus (Fig. 4.3). In patients with a broad rectus abdominis muscle, the lateral part of the muscle may be divided. Using electrocautery, the latissimus dorsi, the external oblique, and the internal oblique muscles are transected, followed by a subperiosteal resection of the anterior part of the 11th rib. The posterior periosteum is incised and the subcostal part of the diaphragm carefully divided, avoiding the neurovascular bundle at the inferior margin of the rib. In the posterior part of the incision, the parietal pleura extends obliquely towards the 12th rib and must be avoided. The transverse abdominal muscle is divided by splitting the fibers and the peritoneum separated from the posterior muscle fascia by blunt dissection. The posterior peritoneal deflection is identified and the renal fascia opened from the pelvic rim to the superior renal pole, except in cases where radical nephrectomy is to be performed.

4.3.1.2
Transverse Abdominal Incision

Transperitoneal access to the kidney by an upper abdominal transverse incision is preferred in uni- or bilateral renal malignancy and in patients where previous renal surgery has been performed through a flank incision. Radical nephrectomy is facilitated by the excellent exposure and the easy access to the renal vessels at an early stage of the operation. The operation is performed with the patient supine. The skin incision starts below the 12th rib, is extended medially parallel to the costal margin at a distance of 2-3 cm, and is then curved horizontally across the midline (Fig. 4.4). The rectus abdominis muscle is transsected. In unilateral renal disease, the incision is extended partly or completely through the rectus muscle on the opposite side. In bilateral renal disease, the incision is extended to the opposite flank. Following transsection of the rectus muscle, the posterior rectus sheath is divided and the peritoneal cavity is carefully entered near the midline. The teres ligament is clamped, divided, and ligated. Lifting the abdominal wall with one hand to avoid intestinal injury, the external and internal oblique and transverse abdominal muscles are divided or separated. The peritoneal cavity is carefully explored to exclude metastasis or any other abnormality. The surgical procedure may be facilitated by using a self-retaining retractor (e.g., Omnitract) to elevate the costal margin(s). A polyethylene intestinal bag may be useful to reduce evaporation and fluid loss from the intestines. The right retrocolic space is entered by incising the peritoneum at its lateral deflection; the ascending colon and the right colonic flexure is then mobilized and displaced medially. Access to the left kidney is obtained by analogous incision of the peritoneum on the left side followed by mobilization of the left colonic flexure and the descending colon.

4.3.1.3
Midline Abdominal Incision

General arteriosclerosis or aneurysm of the aorta and the iliac vessels may require surgical correction in conjunction with renal autotransplantation. A midline abdominal incision (Fig. 4.4) extending from the xiphoid to the pubis provides adequate access to the kidneys as well as the abdominal aorta and the iliac vessels. After incising the linea alba, the peritoneal cavity is entered at the level of the umbilicus. Further dissection of the kidneys is carried out as in the transverse incision.

4.3.2
Nephrectomy for Nonmalignant Disease

An important aspect requiring the surgeon's close attention during the entire procedure is the gentle handling of the kidney. Rough handling, as well as dissection too close to the renal artery, may cause vascular spasm. The resulting decrease in renal perfusion may be followed by acute tubular necrosis (ATN) and delayed graft function after revascularization.

Extensive arterial traction may cause injury to the intima. Pole arteries are especially susceptible, partly due to their small size and partly to the technical difficulty they may create during dissection. Undetected injury may cause arterial thrombosis.

Correct management of the patient during nephrectomy is important for the postoperative graft function. Renal hypoperfusion must be avoided, whether it is caused by systemic arterial hypotension, vascular trauma, or arterial spasm.

Low-molecular heparin, 5000 IU/24 h, is given, starting with 2500 IE preoperatively, to prevent deep venous thrombosis. No extra heparin is added during surgery. Ten to fifteen min prior to nephrectomy 200 ml of mannitol, 150 mg/ml, is administered i.v. to stimulate the diuresis and prevent renal cellular edema (Flores et al. 1972).

In nonmalignant disease, the surgical procedure is identical to the one used in living donor nephrectomy. The opening of Gerota's fascia is followed by identification of the kidney and the renal capsule. The perinephric fat is separated from the kidney by sharp dissection and electrocautery. The plane of dissection must be a few millimeters away from the renal capsule to avoid subcapsular hemorrhage from small retracting capsular vessels. After mobilization of the anterior and posterior surfaces, as well as the superior and inferior poles of the kidney, the ureter and the gonadal vein are identified. Special attention is paid to the ureteral blood supply by avoiding dissection too close to the renal hilar area and by leaving abundant soft tissue around the ureter.

On the left side, the renal vein is identified by following the gonadal vein cranially. The latter is divided close to its junction with the renal vein and ligated using 3–0 absorbable suture. Lumbar tributaries to the renal vein are frequently encountered. In most cases they are easier to divide from the dorsal side of the vein when the dissection of the renal artery is completed, but they may be divided at this stage. Small vessels from the hilar area to the adrenal gland are ligated and divided, thus separating the gland from the kidney. By following the renal vein in a central direction, the suprarenal vein is identified, ligated, and divided. The renal artery is identified, but extensive arterial dissection is avoided at this stage, as it may cause arterial spasm necessitating immediate nephrectomy. The ureter is dissected distally to the level where it crosses the common iliac vessels. Small vessels from the periureteral tissue to the ureter are ligated and divided with careful preservation of abundant periureteral tissue. The use of electrocautery too close to the ureter is avoided as it may create thrombosis of the small vessels responsible for the ureteral blood supply. This may cause ischemic ureteral necrosis and/or strictures. A right-angled clamp is placed on the ureter as far distally as possible, preferably distal to the iliac vessels. The ureter is divided and the distal end ligated using 2–0 absorbable suture.

The final dissection of the renal artery is always carried out as the last part of the surgical procedure. This enables the surgeon to perform immediate nephrectomy if the dissection is followed by renal circulatory disturbances. Leaving some of the perivascular tissue around the artery may prevent arterial spasm, but dissection must be carried out sufficiently close to the artery to enable adequate identification of the vessel and its branches. Extensive traction on the artery must be avoided at any stage, as it may result in disrupture and coiling of the intima. The dissection is carried out down to the aortic wall on the left side. If the suprarenal artery branches off the renal artery, it is ligated and divided.

Clamping and transsection of the renal artery close to the aorta is followed by clamping and transsection of the renal vein. We prefer a long right-angled vascular clamp on the artery. On the left side it is placed close to the aortic wall to obtain maximum arterial length, but sufficient artery must be left to allow safe closure of the artery without injury to the aortic wall. A small exclusion clamp (e.g., Satinsky clamp) is applied to the left renal vein, which then is transsected central to the suprarenal and the gonadal veins.

The central ends of the renal vessels are closed using continuous 5-0 nonabsorbable suture. The artery is further secured with an absorbable ligature, e.g., polyglycolic acid 0 or 1, avoiding traction and injury to the aortic wall.

Nephrectomy of the right kidney is essentially carried out as previously described for the left side. The opening of Gerota's fascia is followed by separation of the perinephric fat from the kidney and complete mobilization of the kidney. The ureter is identified and the gonadal vein, which usually drains directly to the IVC, is retracted medially together with the duodenum, thus achieving access to the anterior and lateral surface of the IVC. The right renal vein, its junction with the IVC, and the adjacent part of the IVC is identified. The adrenal gland is separated from the hilar structures. Isolation and division of the ureter is followed by dissection along the lateral border of the IVC to the renal vein, which is then isolated. At this stage, retraction of the kidney medially permits access to the renal artery, which is then mobilized behind the IVC, but not as far as to the aorta.

The renal artery is then clamped and transsected. A large vascular exclusion clamp is placed on the vena cava, thus allowing the renal vein to be excised with a small patch of the cava (Fig. 4.5). Closure of the defect in the IVC and the renal artery is identical to the closure of the left renal vessels, as already described.

The nephrectomy is followed by meticulous hemostasis using electrocoagulation or ligatures. No postoperative drainage is used. Lateral incisions are closed in a stepwise fashion using a continuous 0 or 1 polyglycolic acid suture in each muscular layer and nonabsorbable skin sutures, interrupted or continuous according to the preference of the surgeon. Transverse incisions may be closed in two or three layers using the same suture material. In midline incisions the fascia is closed using either a double continuous monofilament polyglyconate suture or interrupted polyglycolic acid sutures.

4.3.3
Nephrectomy in Renal Carcinoma

The surgical treatment of renal malignancies is radical nephrectomy with en bloc removal of the kidney, perinephric fat, renal fascia with overlying parietal peritoneum, adrenal gland, and the regional lymph nodes. Likewise, radical nephrectomy is the standard procedure when extracorporeal bench surgery and autotransplantation is considered. When the contralateral adrenal gland has previously been removed, the

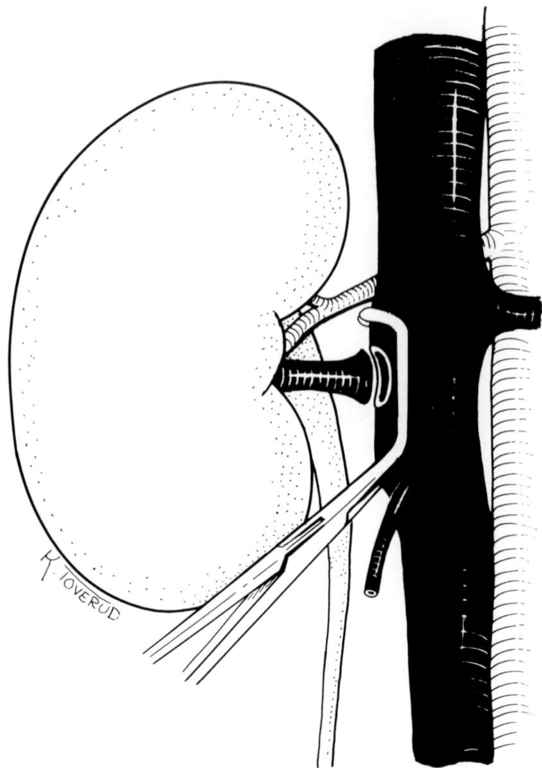

Fig. 4.5. Removal of the right kidney with maximum length of the renal vein

ipsilateral adrenal gland may be left intact whenever this is technically feasible, thus avoiding adrenal insufficiency which may outweigh the potential risk of tumor recurrence. The transabdominal approach is most commonly used. It also allows exploration of the abdominal cavity for metastases. Dissection starts, as previously mentioned, with mobilization of the ipsilateral colon by incising the peritoneum along the avascular lateral deflection and displacing the colon medially. On the right side mobilization of the duodenum (Kocher's maneuver) is performed to allow adequate exposure of the IVC. The central part of the renal vein is identified and isolated, as is the adjacent part of the IVC on the right side. Careful examination of the renal vein at this stage is important, because intraluminal tumor growth excludes autotransplantation and should be followed by early transsection and closure of the renal vessels. The gonadal vein is divided and ligated inferior to the renal pole. On the right side, the gonadal vein is also divided and ligated at its junction with the IVC. The ureter is dissected to the iliac vessels as described in Sect. 4.4.1. In renal malignancy, the ureter is divided inferior to the common iliac vessels and the distal end ligated using absorbable suture. In urothelial malignancies, a complete nephro-ureterectomy is performed. To avoid unnecessary handling of the kidney, the renal artery is approached from the front. On the right side this can be achieved by lifting the renal vein and IVC using, for instance, a small eyelid retractor. The artery can then be isolated behind the IVC, approached either superior or inferior to the renal vein. Isolation of the left renal artery may be difficult until the dissection along the medial border of the adrenal gland is completed. The antero-lateral margin of the aorta is then visible, and the renal artery can be identified and isolated. Mobilization of the kidney is then achieved by careful dissection along the Gerota's fascia in the lateral and posterior part to the level of, or even above, the renal vessels. The extrafascial space is usually traversed by several large veins requiring division between ligatures. Gentle handling is important to minimize the risk of introducing tumor cells into the circulation. The location and size of the tumor may limit the degree of mobilization that can be achieved before transsecting the renal vessels. Tumors situated in the middle or lower part of the kidney usually permit complete mobilization of the kidney before vascular clamping. When the tumor, especially a large one, is situated in the upper pole area of the kidney, the final dissection is usually performed after transsection of the renal vessels. Clamping and division of the renal artery and vein is performed as described previously (Sect. 4.4.1). Dissection is then completed following the Gerota's fascia to the diaphragm, where it is transsected. Special attention is paid to the adrenal vein on the right side to avoid hemorrhage from the vena cava. It is divided between clamps close to the vena cava and ligated. On the left side one or several large veins superior to the adrenal gland usually need to be divided. The kidney with perinephric fat, renal fascia, and adrenal gland can then be removed for extracorporeal preservation and surgery. Remaining regional lymph nodes are carefully dissected and removed for histopathological examination. Closure of the vessels and the wound is performed as described in Sect. 4.4.1.

4.4
Extracorporeal Renal Preservation

Renal tissue is sensitive to normothermic ischemia (warm ischemia). A warm ischemia time (WIT) of about 20 min is generally acceptable, but 30 min or more WIT is distinctly deleterious (Grundmann et al. 1979). Perfusion and preservation techniques have evolved in the renal allotransplantation era allowing cold storage of kidneys for more than 48 h.

Hypothermia is the basic principle of the preservation techniques presently used, either as simple hypothermic storage or as continuous hypothermic perfusion (Toledo-Pereyra and Rodriquez 1994). Kidneys subjected to less than 15 min WIT can be preserved effectively up to 30 h by a brief intraarterial flush immediately after removal, using a chilled (5-10°C) hypertonic solution, (e.g., Euro-Collins solution) followed by storage at 5-10°C (Jacobsen and Pegg 1981). This is more than adequate for extracorporeal renal surgery, where the preservation time usually does not exceed a few hours. The method is inexpensive and simple compared to continuous hypothermic perfusion (Jacobsen and Pegg 1981), which under these circumstances offers no advantages.

Immediately after nephrectomy, the kidney is placed in a basin containing cold saline. The renal artery is cannulated using a soft polyethylene tube or infusion

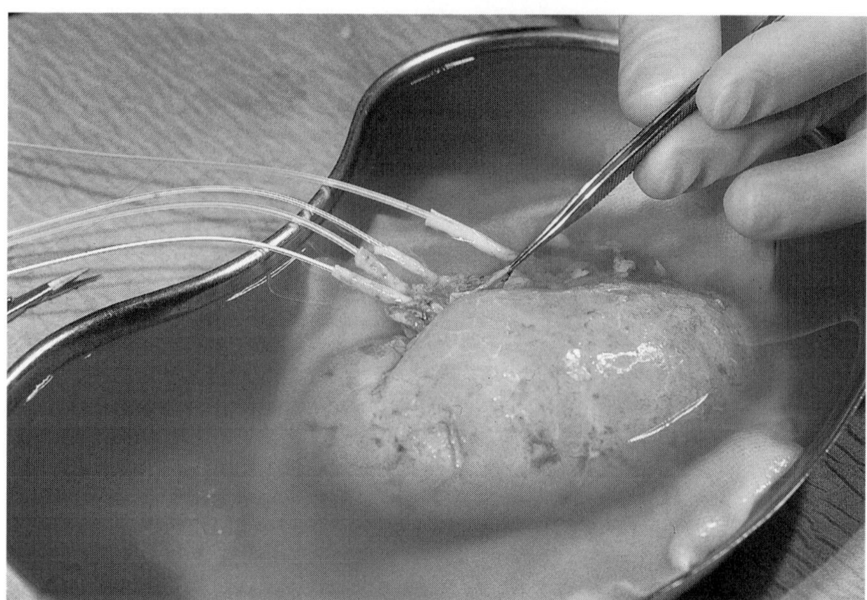

Fig. 4.6. Perfusion of the kidney with chilled (5-10°C) Euro-Collins solution immediately after nephrectomy. Observe the four separate arteries of this kidney

cannula, the size being determined by the diameter of the artery, usually 6-10 F. The kidney is flushed with Euro-Collins solution at about 5-10°C (Fig. 4.6). Any other currently used preservation fluids may of course replace Euro-Collins solution, but will usually be more expensive and offer no advantages regarding graft function (Toledo-Pereyra and Rodriguez 1994). Solutions for i.v. purposes (e.g., Ringer's lactate) should not be used for preservation times exceeding 3 h (Jacobsen and Pegg 1981). Heparin is not added to the perfusate. Finger pressure is sufficient to hold the cannula in place. Flushing is carried out with a perfusion pressure of 100-150 cm H_2O, and is continued until the efflux from the renal vein is clear and the kidney has a pale yellow-white color. This usually requires about 200-500 ml of perfusate. Elevation of the perfusion pressure is of no advantage, as experimental studies indicate that a high perfusion pressure (60 mm Hg) causes more endothelial damage than low pressure (30 mm Hg) (Cerra et al. 1977). There is also evidence that too rapid cooling may be damaging per se (Jacobsen et al. 1979; Francavilla et al. 1973). During the subsequent bench surgery, the kidney is kept in the basin in cold saline. A stable low temperature is obtained by adding frozen cubes of saline during the procedure. Covering the ice with sponges prevents direct contact between the ice and kidney. During the transplantation, the kidney is packed in chilled sponges, which are frequently changed to keep the temperature down (see Chap. 5).

References

Cerra FB, Raza S, Andres GA, Siegel JH (1977) The endothelial damage of pulsatile renal preservation and its relationship to perfusion pressure and colloid osmotic pressure. Surgery 81:534-541

Dyson M (1995) Urinary system. In: Bannister LH et al. (eds) Gray's Anatomy. Churchill Livingstone, Edinburgh, pp 1815-1827

Flores J, DiBona DR, Beck CH, Leaf A (1972) The role of cell swelling in ischaemic renal damage and the protective effect of hypertonic solute. J Clin Invest 51:118-126

Francavilla A, Brown TH, Fiore R, Cascardo S, Taylor P, Groth CG (1973) Preservation of organs for transplantation. Evidence of detrimental effect of rapid cooling. Eur Surg Res 5:384-389

Grundmann R, Bischoff A, Albrod A, Pichlmaier H (1979) Canine kidney perfusion after various warm ischemic periods. In: Pegg DE, Jacobsen IA (eds) Organ preservation II. Churchill Livingstone, Edinburgh, pp 33-45

Jacobsen IA, Kemp E, Buhl MR (1979) An adverse effect of rapid cooling in kidney preservation. Transplantation 27:135-136

Jacobsen IA, Pegg DE (1981) Organ preservation. Kidney. In: Karow AM, Pegg DE (eds) Organ preservation for transplantation. Marcel Dekker, New York, pp 553-576

Marshall FF (1986) Anatomy of the retroperitoneum. In: Walsh PC et al. (eds) Campbell's Urology. Saunders, Philadelphia, pp 2-11

Olsson C A (1986) Anatomy of the upper urinary tract. In: Walsh PC et al. (eds) Campbell's Urology. Saunders, Philadelphia, pp 12-46

Perlmutter AD, Retik AB, Baure SB (1986) Anomalies of the upper urinary tract. In: Walsh PC et al. (eds) Campbell's Urology. Saunders, Philadelphia, pp 1665-1759

Toledo-Pereyra LH, Rodriguez FJ (1994) Scientific basis and current status of organ preservation. Transplant Proc 26(1):309-311

Renal Autotransplantation: Indications, Basic Surgical Techniques, and Complications

Inge B. Brekke and Gunnar Sødal

5.1
Introduction and Historical Background

The demonstration provided by the initial allotransplantations performed in the 1950s that renal transplantation is technically feasible raised the prospects for extracorporeal renal repair and subsequent autotransplantation. In 1963, high ureteral injury was managed by kidney autotransplantation (Hardy 1963), and in 1967, extracorporeal repair of an occluded renal artery and autotransplantation of the kidney was performed by Ota (Ota et al. 1967). The development of organ preservation techniques allowed prolonged reversible ischemia. In 1971, Gelin and associates reported on ex vivo renal preservation during bench surgery lasting several hours (Gelin et al. 1971).

Since then, renal autotransplantation has become a valid alternative to in situ methods, primarily being used by renal transplant surgeons for the treatment of various renovascular or urological conditions (Belzer et al. 1970; Dubernard et al. 1985; Flatmark et al. 1989; Novick et al. 1990). Preservation perfusates and extracorporeal cold storage of the kidney make extensive and time consuming repair work on renal parenchyma, renal arteries, ureter, and pelvis possible without jeopardizing kidney function through ischemic damage. Ex vivo surgery may thus be used to salvage kidneys in a number of patients where the alternative would be nephrectomy (Fowl et al. 1986). In extreme cases, cold storage of the kidney may even allow for the replantation to be postponed to the next day, to await circulatory stabilization of an unstable patient (Campbell et al. 1993).

The decision whether in situ or ex vivo surgery should be chosen for a patient with a renal artery abnormality or urologic disorder must first of all be based on the complexity of the planned treatment, but also on the preference and experience of the surgeon. The restricted exposure obtainable with in situ surgery and the limits of tolerable associated warm ischemia can result in kidney failure due to nonoptimal repair and/or ischemic damage. Therefore, the more complex renal lesions are better treated by extracorporeal repair, during hypothermia, on a side table, performed under optimal conditions that allows for meticulous repair work and followed by autotransplantation.

From 1973 to 1994, 502 renal autotransplantations were performed in our renal transplant unit for various indications. The technical details and results of these cases are described in the following chapters. For the preoperative work-up, see Chaps. 2 and 3.

5.2
Indications

Renal autotransplantation with or without extracorporeal repair is a logical option in a variety of conditions. The most frequent indications have been renal artery disease (Novick 1984; Flatmark et al. 1989; Brekke et al. 1992; Brunetti et al. 1994; Murray et al. 1994), urological disorders (Bondevik et al. 1990; Novick et al. 1990 ; Lindblad et al. 1993; Rembrink et al. 1993), including renal (Stormont et al. 1992; van der Velden et al. 1992), pelvic, or ureteral neoplasms (Pettersson et al. 1981). Other indications have been aortic aneurysm (Adib and Belzer 1978; Cameron et al. 1982; Mohr and Sødal 1980; Spanos et al. 1974), chronic hematuria (Sheil et al. 1987; Qunibi 1988), retroperitoneal fibrosis (Rose et al. 1984; Mikkelsen and Lepor 1989), and idiopathic chyluria (Brunkwall et al. 1989). Autotransplantation of a kidney to a site outside the radiation field has likewise been reported as a kidney-saving procedure before radiotherapy (Hitchcock et al. 1993).

Extracorporeal renal vascular reconstruction and autotransplantation has also contributed to improved outcome in pediatric patients with renovascular hypertension (RVH) and can be performed in children even less than 1 year of age (Jordan et al. 1985; Tapper et al. 1986). For the most common indications, details on the selection of patients, preoperative considerations, and results, see Chaps. 6-11.

5.3
Basic Surgical Techniques

When the patient is anesthetized, a large-bore Foley catheter is inserted and the bladder is irrigated with a neomycin sulfate solution. A non-nephrotoxic, broad spectrum antibiotic is given as perioperative antibacterial prophylaxis. Depending on the indication for surgery, the patient is initially positioned on the side or supine on the operating table, and nephrectomy is done through a flank or midline incision. A detailed description of the particulars to be considered at nephrectomy is given in Chap. 4.

5.3.1
Extracorporeal Preparation of the Kidney

Hypothermia is the cornerstone of extracorporeal organ repair. Cooling of the renal parenchyma to 10°C reduces the renal metabolism to less than 5% of normal (Semb et al. 1960), allowing several hours of ischemia.

Following nephrectomia, the kidney is flushed with a cold electrolyte solution (see Chap. 4). Preparatory surgery is then performed with the kidney in a basin with ice slush. When this has been performed as described in the following chapters, reimplantation of the kidney is prepared. Removal of some of the perinephric fat surrounding the kidney and dissection of the renal vessels will ease the implantation of the kidney, but the dissection should not be carried unnecessarily far into the hilar region, where small vascular branches are easily injured. As there is no collateral arterial supply within the kidney, preservation of all arteries and branches is mandatory to prevent infarction of renal segments. Accessory arteries or branches to the inferior

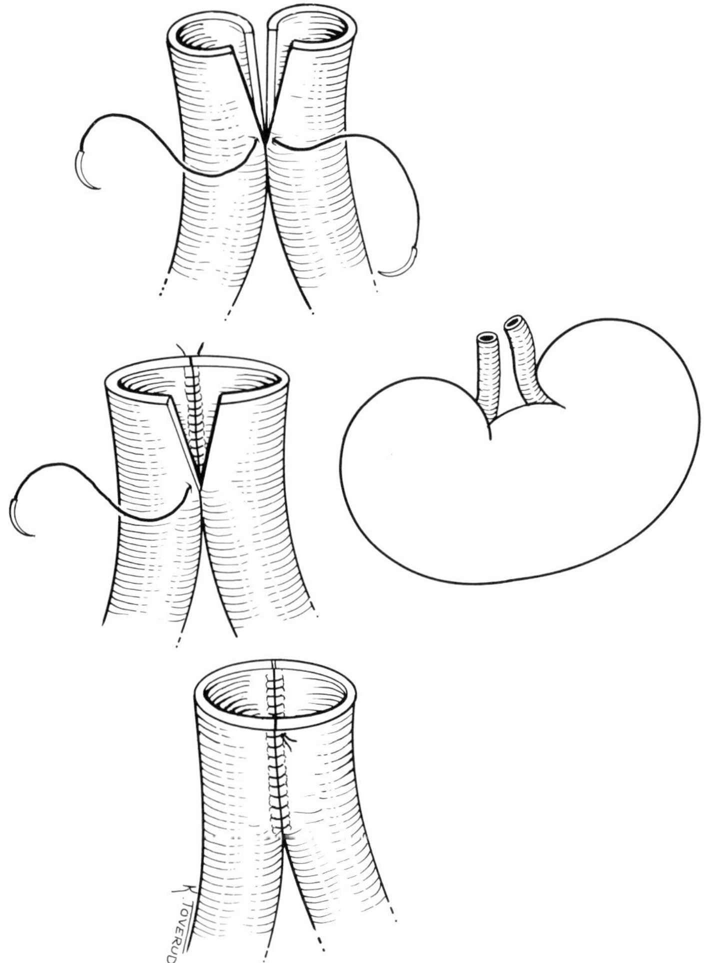

Fig. 5.1. Accessory renal arteries joined by the „double barrel technique"

pole are especially important for the blood supply of the ureter. Failure to preserve these arteries may cause ureteral necrosis and urine leak or fibrosis and obstruction.

Multiple renal arteries have been shown to be present in 25%-30% of kidneys (Anson et al. 1936; Boijsen 1959). Two arteries of equal length may be joined by the „double barrel technique" to form a common orifice (Fig. 5.1). When one artery is considerably shorter than the other, the shorter artery may be anastomosed to the side of the larger artery (Fig. 5.2). In the case of other arterial abnormalities, special reconstructive procedures have to be considered and grafts may be used to substitute for renal artery segments or branches (Fig. 5.3) (see also Chap. 7).

Numerous collaterals present on the venous side allow in the vast majority of cases nondominant renal veins to be ligated without impairing renal venous drainage (Pick and Anson 1940).

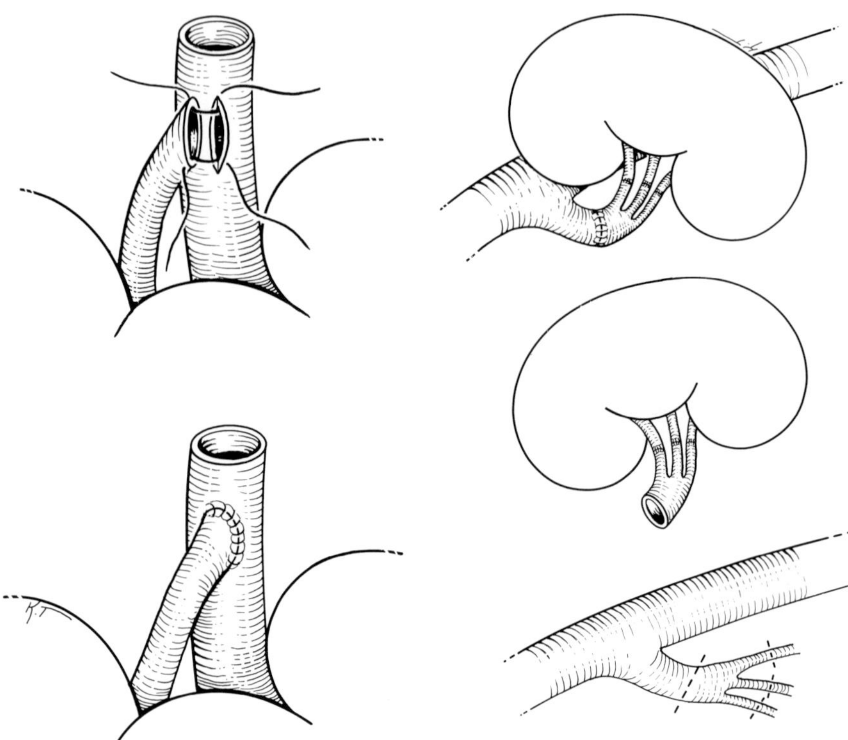

Fig. 5.2. Accessory renal artery anastomosed end-to-side to the main artery

Fig. 5.3. Renal artery reconstruction using autogenous internal iliac artery graft

5.3.2
Kidney Replantation

The principal technique of renal autotransplantation does not differ from that of renal allotransplantation (Salmela et al. 1995), only vascular and ureteral reconstructions require some extra considerations.

The preferred site for renal placement is the iliac fossa with vascular anastomoses to the iliac vessels. The topographic relationships of the renal pelvis and renal vessels should be considered when choosing the recipient side. Placing the right kidney on the left side and vice versa makes access to the renal pelvis easier for a possible intervention in the postoperative period. When one kidney is autotransplanted and the contralateral kidney is left in situ, the autograft should preferably be placed on the side opposite the in situ kidney. Otherwise the autograft may cause obstruction of the in situ ureter.

In older patients, however, it may be more important to chose the side with the least atherosclerotic iliac arteries or the side opposite to a previous lower extremity vein thrombosis, which may have left an occluded iliac vein. For these reasons, if the nephrectomy has been performed through a midline incision, the iliac vessels should

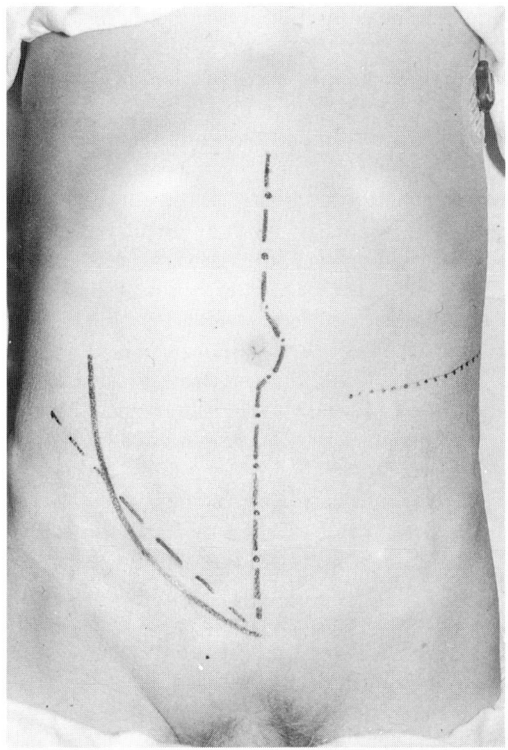

Fig. 5.4. Alternative incisions for nephrectomy and graft implantation

be inspected and palpated. In most cases, a preoperative angiography will be useful in deciding which iliac fossa should be preferred. If there is doubt about the patency of the iliac veins, ultrasound or venography may be performed preoperatively. When, during the operation, the external iliac vein is found inadequate for renal outflow, a renal venous anastomosis to the common iliac vein or caval vein is a valid alternative.

If the nephrectomy has been performed through a midline incision, transplantation may be carried out through the same incision. However, this may give less satisfactory access to the iliac vessels, especially in obese male patients.

If the kidney has been removed through a flank incision, the wound is closed and the patient is placed in the supine position. A semilunar skin incision is made in the lower abdominal quadrant, extending from the midline to above the anterior superior iliac spine (Fig. 5.4). The external oblique, internal oblique, and transversus abdominis muscles are divided. The inferior epigastric vessels are identified lateral to the rectus muscle, ligated, and divided. In the female patient, the round ligament is ligated and cut. In the male patient, the spermatic cord is retracted medially or, in older patients, ligated and cut if necessary for optimal exposure of the iliac vessels. Extraperitoneal access to the iliac vessels is obtained by pushing the peritoneum cranially.

A self-retaining retractor is inserted to facilitate exposure of the operative field (Fig. 5.5). The lateral blade of the retractor is padded to avoid injury to the lateral femoral cutaneous nerve (Vaziri et al. 1976), while care is taken to avoid compression of the common iliac artery by the cranial blade.

The entire external iliac vein is mobilized, and tributaries, when present, are ligated and cut. All overlying lymphatic tissue is ligated with absorbable 3/0 to 5/0 suture to avoid postoperative lymphocele formation. If the renal vein is extremely short, the internal iliac vein may be divided to allow more extensive mobilization of the external iliac vein and thus ease the suturing of the venous anastomosis, but special care must be taken in securing the cut end of the internal iliac vein. Slipping of a ligature will cause bleeding that may be difficult to control.

Unlike the cadaveric renal graft, the autotransplant has no aortic patch, so most surgeons will prefer to perform an end-to-end anastomosis to the internal iliac artery. One should, however, avoid bilateral use of the internal artery because this may impair the blood supply to the gluteal muscles and cause impotence in the male patient (Flanigan et al. 1982). The internal iliac artery is mobilized from its origin to, or past, its branches. The branches are ligated and the internal iliac artery is cut distally after a clamp has been placed proximally. Placing the ligature proximal to the branches, at the trunk of the internal iliac artery, and thus leaving the branches intact (Fig. 5.5), may be of importance for the pelvic collateral circulation. Atherosclerotic plaques are removed through the cut end of the artery or, if more extensive atherosclerosis is present, an endarterectomy of the entire artery may be performed through a common iliac arteriotomy. If occluded by atherosclerosis, as is common in older patients, the external iliac or common iliac artery may be selected for an end-to-side anastomosis, choosing the segment with the least atherosclerosis. A local endarterectomy is performed when necessary.

When the recipient artery and vein are prepared, clamps are placed at the cranial and caudal end of the external iliac vein, and a venotomy is adjusted to the diameter of the renal vein. Occasionally, a valve may be seen beneath or at the venotomy site. If the valve is likely to interfere with the anastomosis it should be carefully excised. The external iliac vein and internal iliac artery are flushed with heparin solution. Stay sutures are placed at both ends of the venotomy, and a third suture at the medial venotomy lip (Fig. 5.5).

The kidney is then placed in the operative field packed in chilled sponges and the end-to-side anastomosis to the external iliac vein is finished with continuous sutures. The renal vein is clamped and the clamps on the external iliac vein are removed, starting with the proximal clamp, reestablishing venous blood flow from the lower extremity.

When the venous anastomosis is patent, the renal artery is anastomosed to the selected artery. Both anastomoses are performed with continuous 6/0 prolene sutures, placing the knots a few millimeters away from the vessel wall to allow for some lumen expansion or „growth factor „ (Starzl et al. 1984) when releasing the blood flow through the vessels. Alternatively, if the renal artery has a small diameter, the arterial anastomosis is performed with interrupted sutures in one or both halves of the circumference. The relative shortness of the right renal vein compared to the artery may increase the risk of artery kinking. This risk is reduced by shortening the artery before making the anastomosis. Furosemid, 40 mg, is given intravenously a few minutes be-

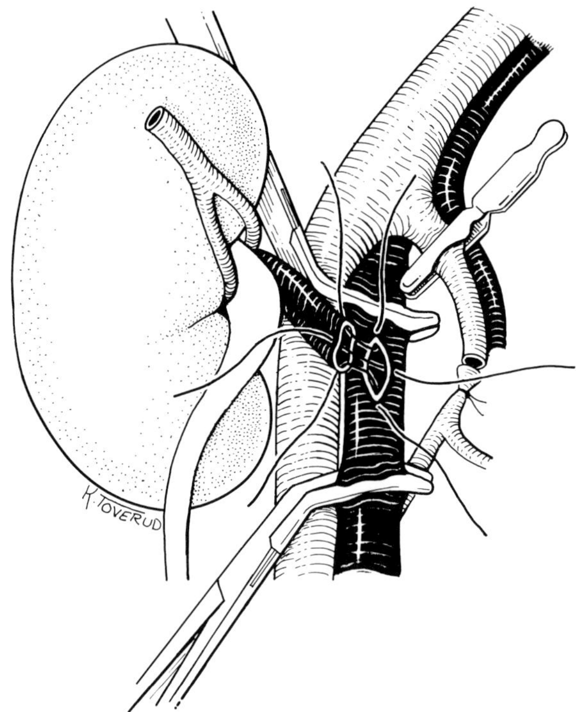

Fig. 5.5. Kidney reimplantation. The internal iliac artery is ligated and transected distally. The external iliac vein is clamped. A venotomy of a length appropriate for the diameter of the renal vein is made, and three stay sutures are inserted

fore revascularization, and 200 ml of 20% mannitol solution is infused when diuresis has started.

Ureteroneocystostomy is preferred for urinary tract reconstruction based on the low complication rate associated with this method, compared to ureteroureterostomy or ureteropyelostomy (Salvatierra et al. 1977). In cases of neoplasms involving the ureter, the ureter is resected and a pyelocystostomy is performed (see Chaps. 8 and 9). To help identify the bladder, bladder distention is obtained by clamping the urethral catheter some time in advance to allow for urine to fill the bladder, or when no urine is produced, by instillation of 150-200 cc sterile saline through the catheter. Two stay sutures are placed in the bladder wall and the bladder is opened through an anterior transverse cystostomy. The incision is preferably made with electrocautery to prevent bleeding from the well vascularized bladder wall. Retractors are placed into the lumen. The ureter is passed under the spermatic cord and through a separate stab incision in the bladder wall (Fig. 5.6A), care being taken to avoid ureteral twisting. After having shortened the ureter to a suitable length, the ureteral end is spatulated for a distance of 1-1.5 cm and anastomosed to the bladder mucosa with interrupted 5/0 absorbable suture. Various modifications of the Politano-Leadbetter method (Politano and Leadbetter 1958) may be used. Our preferred technique is that described by Paquin (1959), which includes passing the ureter through a 2 cm submucosal tunnel (Fig. 5.6B) before

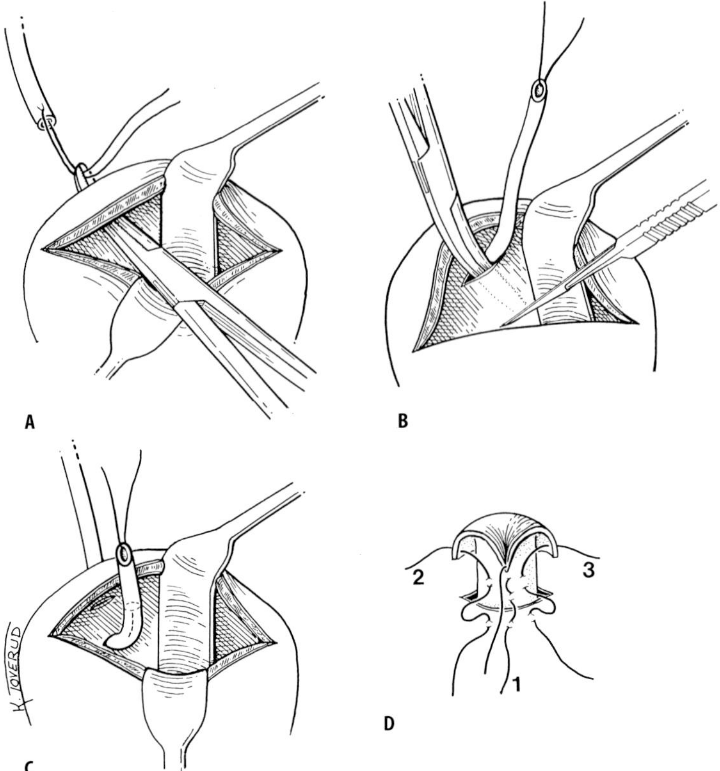

Fig. 5.6A-D. A stab incision is made in the posterolateral part of the bladder via a transverse cystostomy. The ureter is brought through the stab incision (A) and through a submucosal tunnel (B and C) before fashioning the ureteral nipple (D)

performing the anastomosis to the bladder (Fig. 5.6C and D). If the passage of urine is not observed, an 8 F catheter or feeding tube may be inserted through the ureter to the pelvis to rule out stenotic parts. When any obstruction is suspected, the catheter may be left as a stent in the ureter and brought out in the suprapubic area; otherwise, it is removed before closing the bladder. If the stent is left in place, the passage through the ureter is easily examined postoperatively by pyelography.

To avoid the risk of complications related to a ureteral implantation, some surgeons prefer to leave the ureter intact during nephrectomy and perform the extraperitoneal repair work in a basin on the abdomen of the patient (Dubernard et al. 1985; Dean and Hansen 1990; Murray et al. 1994). In this way an orthotopic autotransplantation back into the renal fossa can be performed. However, to some degree, the advantages of ex vivo bench surgery after complete removal of the kidney and the excellent working conditions it offers at the side table are then lost. Furthermore, with the kidney on a side table the patient can be taken care of by a second team of surgeons, the nephrectomy incision closed, and the recipient site prepared for the transplantation of the kidney.

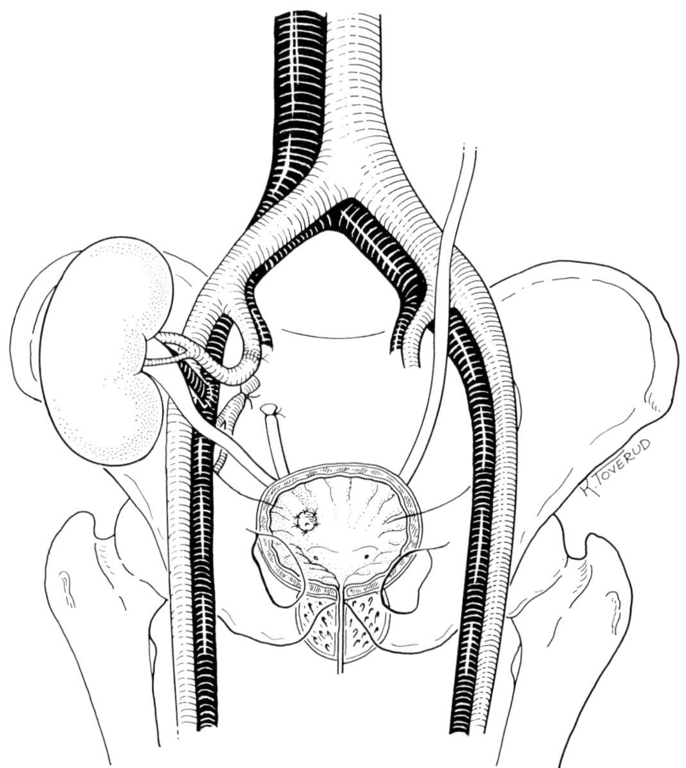

Fig. 5.7. Sketch showing the position of the autotransplanted kidney in the iliac fossa

After closing the cystostomy by absorbable sutures in 2-3 layers, the autotransplant is positioned in the pelvis. The standard position is with the kidney on the psoas muscle and the hilum directed medially or somewhat caudally (Fig. 5.7). When positioning the kidney, however, care must be taken to place the kidney in a position that prevents kinking of the renal artery, especially after extensive vascular reconstruction or when multiple renal arteries are present.

When bench surgery has been performed on renal parenchyma or pelvis, a suction drain is usually placed along the graft before the wound is closed in two muscle layers with absorbable suture, followed by skin closure.

A bladder catheter is left for 2-3 days. Thrombosis prophylaxis with subcutaneously administered low molecular weight heparin is started preoperatively and continued until the patient is fully mobilized.

5.4
Complications

The surgical complications associated with renal autotransplantation will be of the same categories as those following renal allografting (Plainfosse et al. 1992; Amante and Kahan 1994). In addition, extracorporeal surgery will have a potential for various complications, depending on the type of bench surgery performed. On the other hand, recipients of autografts are not exposed to the hazards of immunosuppression and, due to its usually shorter ischemia time, the autograft is less prone to ischemic damage with tubular necrosis. In contrast to our experience with renal allotransplantation, a lymphocele was seen in only one of the patients who underwent renal autotransplantation.

Renal artery stenosis caused by atherosclerosis may be considered an independent marker for coronary artery disease (CAD) (Valentine et al. 1993), and CAD is a major cause of morbidity and mortality after surgery for RVH. This has to be considered in the preoperative work-up, with stress on diagnosing serious CAD, which should then be given therapeutic preference.

5.4.1
Vascular Complications

The most common complications in any vascular procedure are hemorrhage and thrombosis (Dodd et al. 1991). Perioperative hemorrhages are most often from the vascular anastomoses or from branches that have been overseen during bench surgery. Serious bleeding from the venous anastomosis seldom occurs at the time of revascularization, because of the low venous blood pressure, and minor bleeding will stop after a few minutes. Larger volumes of blood may be lost through unligated left renal vein branches, i.e., suprarenal, gonadal, and lumbar branches. These are usually easily managed by a few stitches. A larger arterial anastomosal bleeding may be more difficult to control, especially when calcified atheromatous plaques are present at or near the suture line in the iliac artery. Occasionally, autotransplant repeat perfusion with chilled Ringer's acetate and arterial anastomosis re-do may be required.

Sluggish renal reperfusion may be caused by renal artery spasm, stenosis at the site of anastomosis, or kinking (Frauchiger et al. 1994). Vasospasm usually vanishes after 10-30 min. The beneficial effect of calcium channel blockers on renal microcirculation (Epstein 1993) may be utilized to prevent vasospasm by giving 20 mg of nifedipin sublingually or 1.25 mg of verapamil directly into the renal artery.

Arterial kinking is usually caused by a too long renal artery or malplacement of the anastomosis. If the kinking is not correctable by positioning of the kidney, redoing the anastomosis must be considered. If the anastomosis itself is satisfactory, the easiest and safest method of shortening the artery or correcting a twist is to cut the arterial trunk, shorten or de-twist the artery, and reunite the ends by an end-to-end anastomosis. Peroperative ultrasonic-Doppler arterial flow measurements will show whether the result is satisfactory.

5.4.2
Urologic Complications

When attention is paid to the technical details described above, urologic complications following renal autotransplantation are quite rare. The most common complications are leaks and ureteral obstruction (Dreikorn 1992).

Urine leaks are very rare when ureteral reimplantation is performed by the Paquin or similar methods, and the bladder is closed in 2-3 layers. An incorrectly closed cystostomy or a disrupted ureterocystostomy are the most frequent sites of a leak. Surgical reintervention is usually required to solve the problem. Urinary leaks through nephrotomies made during removal of renal concrements or from the resection site after excision of a neoplasm are quite commonly seen and are drained through suction drains until the leakage subsides after a few days.

Obstruction of urinary flow is often a more difficult task to handle. An obstruction will often cause a rise in creatinine and may be confirmed by an ultrasound examination showing expansion of the renal pelvis. In the presence of a well functioning contralateral kidney, however, there may be no significant rise in creatinine. Therefore, it is always advisable to perform at least one ultrasound examination in the first postoperative week. When a distended pelvis is shown by ultrasound, it must be decided whether there is a real obstruction affecting the autograft function. If in doubt, excretory renography and isotope renography will give further information. If no functional impairment can be diagnosed, the patient is followed with frequent ultrasound and creatinine controls for 2-3 months to ensure stable autograft function. Routines for further follow-up are given in Chaps. 6-11.

The site of an obstruction is most often at the distal end of the ureter, at the nipple, or in the part of the ureter that passes through the bladder wall. The ureteral orifice may be obstructed by a blood clot, by edema of the created nipple, by a falsely placed suture, or the ureter may be twisted. Late obstruction may sometimes be the result of ureteral fibrosis caused by impaired blood supply to the distal ureter.

When a functionally significant obstruction is diagnosed, two therapeutic alternatives must be considered. A partial obstruction may be treated by the insertion of a double-J catheter, either retrograde through a cystoscope or antegrade through a percutaneous nephrostomy. A significant stenosis diagnosed in the early postoperative course is better dealt with by surgery, usually meaning re-doing the ureterocystostomy.

Lymphoceles, which occur in 5%-18% of cases after renal allotransplantation and often cause ureteral obstruction (Khauli et al. 1993; Øyen et al. 1995), seem to be extremely rare after autotransplantation; only one has been seen in our series of 502 autotransplanted kidneys. This may indicate that the immunosuppressive therapy, imperative for allograft survival, plays a role in the development of lymphoceles.

References

Adib K, Belzer FO (1978) Renal autotransplantation in dissecting aortic aneurysm with renal artery involvement. Surgery 84(5):686-688

Amante AJ, Kahan BD (1994) Technical complications of renal transplantation. Surg Clin North Am 74(5):1117-1131

Anson BJ, Richardson GA, Minear WL (1936) Variations in the number and arrangement of the renal vessels: study of the blood supply of 400 kidneys. J Urol 36:211-219

Belzer FO, Keaveny TV, Reed TW, Pryor JP (1970) A new method of renal artery reconstruction. Surgery 68(4):619-624

Boijsen E (1959) Angiographic studies of the anatomy of single and multiple renal arteries. Acta Radiol Suppl 183:1-135

Bondevik H, Albrechtsen D, Sodal G, Jakobsen A, Brekke I, Flatmark A (1990) Extracorporeal surgery and autotransplantation for complicated renal calculous disease in 108 kidneys. Scand J Urol Nephrol 24(4): 301-306

Brekke I B, Sødal G, Jakobsen A, Bentdal O, Pfeffer P, Albrechtsen D, Flatmark A (1992) Fibro-muscular renal artery disease treated by extracorporeal vascular reconstruction and renal autotransplantation: short- and long-term results. Eur J Vasc Surg 6(5):471-476

Brunetti DR, Sasaki TM, Friedlander G, Edson M, Harviel JD, Adams WD, Ghaseiman R, Cabellon SJ (1994) Successful renal autotransplantation in a patient with bilateral renal artery thrombosis. Urology 43(2):235-237

Brunkwall J, Simonsen O, Bergqvist D, Jonsson K, Bergentz SE (1989) Massive idiopathic chyluria treated by autotransplantation (in Swedish). Läkartidningen 86(28-29):2533-2534

Cameron AE, Graham JC, Hamilton WA, O'Neal H, Rudge CJ, Bewick M, Cotton LT (1982) Suprarenal aortic aneurysm: an unsuccessful attempt at renal autotransplantation. Angiology 33(12):806-810

Campbell SC, Gill I, Novick AC (1993) Delayed allograft autotransplantation after excision of a large symptomatic renal artery pseudoaneurysm. J Urol 149(2):361-363

Dean RH, Hansen KJ (1990) "Re-do" procedures after failed angioplasty or renovascular operation, and ex-vivo repairs. In: Bergan JJ, Yao JST (eds) Techniques in arterial surgery. Saunders, Philadelphia

Dodd G, Tublin ME, Shah A, Zajko AB (1991) Imaging of vascular complications associated with renal transplants. AJR 157(3): 449-459

Dreikorn K (1992) Problems of the distal ureter in renal transplantation (Review). Urol Int 49(2):76-89

Dubernard JM, Martin X, Mongin D, Gelet A, Canton F (1985) Extracorporeal replacement of the renal artery: techniques, indications and long-term results. J Urol 133(1):13-16

Epstein M (1993) Calcium antagonists and the kidney. Implications for renal protection. Am J Hypertens. 6:251-259

Flanigan DP, Schuler JJ, Keifer T, Schwartz JA, Lim LT (1982) Elimination of iatrogenic impotence and improvement of sexual function after aortoiliac revascularization. Arch Surg 117(5):544-550

Flatmark A, Albrechtsen D, Sodal G, Bondevik H, Jakobsen A Jr, Brekke IB (1989) Renal autotransplantation. World J Surg 13(2):206-209

Fowl RJ, Hollier LH, Bernatz PE, Pairolero PC, Vogt PA, Cherry KJ (1986) Repeat revascularization versus nephrectomy in the treatment of recurrent renovascular hypertension. Surg Gynecol Obstet 162(1):37-42

Frauchiger B, Bock A, Spoendlin M, Eichlisberger R, Vogelbach P, Landmann J, Thiel G, Jager K (1994) Early renal transplant dysfunction due to arterial kinking stenosis. Nephrol Dial Transplant 9(1):76-79

Gelin LE, Claes G, Gustafsson A, Storm B (1971) Total bloodlessness for extracorporeal organ repair. Rev Surg 28(5):305-316

Hardy JD (1963) High ureteral injury: management by autotransplantation of the kidney. JAMA 184: 97-101

Hitchcock R, Kohler J, Duffy PG, Malone PS (1993) Renal autotransplantation - a kidney saving procedure before spinal radiotherapy. Pediatr Hematol Oncol 10(4):333-335

Jordan ML, Novick AC, Cunningham RL (1985) The role of renal autotransplantation in pediatric and young adult patients with renal artery disease. J Vasc Surg 2(3):385-392

Khauli RB, Stoff JS, Lovewell T, Ghavamian R, Baker S (1993) Post-transplant lymphoceles: a critical look into the risk factors, pathophysiology and management. J Urol 150(1):22-26

Lindblad B, Bergqvist D, Kristiansen P (1993) Bilateral renal autotransplantation with direct pyelocystostomy in a patient with frequent disabling nephroureterolithiasis. Case report. Scand J Urol Nephrol 27(3):413-414

Mikkelsen D, Lepor H (1989) Innovative surgical management of idiopathic retroperitoneal fibrosis. J Urol 141(5):1192-1196

Mohr E, Sødal G (1980) Aorto-enteric fistula. A case treated with insertion of a new dacron prosthesis and bilateral autotransplantation of the kidneys. Scand J Thorac Cardiovasc Surg 14(1):97-99

Murray SP, Kent C, Salvatierra O, Stoney RJ (1994) Complex branch renovascular disease: management options and late results. J Vasc Surg 20(3):338-345

Novick AC (1984) Microvascular reconstruction of complex branch renal artery disease. Urol Clin North Am 11(3):465-475

Novick AC, Jackson CL, Straffon RA (1990) The role of renal autotransplantation in complex urological reconstruction. J Urol 143(3):452-457

Ota K, Mori S, Awane Y, Ueno A (1967) Ex situ repair of renal artery for renovascular hypertension. Arch Surg 94(3):370-373

Øyen O, Bakka A, Pfeffer P, Foss A, Bentdal Ø, Jørgensen P, Brekke IB, Sødal G (1995) Laparoscopic management of posttransplant pelvic lymphoceles. Transplant Proc 27(6):3449

Paquin AJ (1959) Ureterovesical anastomosis. The description and evaluation of a technique. J Urol 82:573-583

Pettersson S, Brynger H, Johansson S, Nilson AE (1981) Extracorporeal kidney surgery and calicovesicostomy in urothelial tumors of the upper urinary tract (in German). Z Urol Nephrol 74(2):113-118

Pick JW, Anson BJ (1940) The renal vascular pedicle: an anatomical study of 430 body-halves. J Urol 44:411-434

Plainfosse MC, Calonge VM, Beyloune MC, Glotz D, Duboust A (1992) Vascular complications in the adult kidney transplant recipient. J Clin Ultrasound 20(8):517-527

Politano VA, Leadbetter WF (1958) An operative technique for the correction of vesicoureteral reflux. J Urol 79(6):932-941

Qunibi WY (1988) Renal autotransplantation for severe sickle cell haematuria (letter). Lancet 1(8579):236-237

Rembrink K, Niebel W, Behrendt H (1993) Autotransplantation of the kidney. Indications and results (in German). Urologe A 32(2):151-155

Rose MC, Novick AC, Rybka SJ (1984) Renal autotransplantation in patients with retroperitoneal fibrosis. Cleve Clin Q 51(2):357-363

Salmela K, Ahonen J, Kootstra G (1995) Renal transolantation. In: Harjula A, Höckerstedt K (eds) Atlas of clinical transplantation. Jyväskylä, Recallmed

Salvatierra OJ, Olcott C, Amend WJ, Cochrum KC, Freduska NJ (1977) Urological complications of renal transplantation can be prevented or controlled. J Urol 117(4):421-424

Semb G, Krog J, Johansen K (1960) Renal metabolism and blood flow during local hypothermia: studies by means of renal perfusion in situ. Acta Chir Scand Suppl 253:196-202

Sheil AG, Ibels LS, Pollock C, Graham JC, Short J (1987) Treatment of loin pain/haematuria syndrome by renal autotransplantation (letter). Lancet 2(8564):907-908

Spanos PK, Mozes MM, Najarian JS (1974) Resection of suprarenal aortic aneurysm with autotransplantation of the kidney. Ann Surg 180(6):823-826

Starzl TE, Iwatsuki S, Shaw BW (1984) A growth factor in fine vascular anastomoses. Surg Gynecol Obstet 159:164-165

Stormont TJ, Bilhartz DL, Zincke H (1992) Pitfalls of „bench surgery" and autotransplantation for renal cell carcinoma. Mayo Clin Proc 67(7):621-628

Tapper D, Brand T, Burns M, Hickman R (1986) Technical consideration in management of renovascular hypertension in an infant with double renal arteries. J Pediatr Surg 21(12):1064-1067

Valentine RJ, Clagett GP, Miller GL, Myers SI, Martin JD, Chervu A (1993) The coronary risk of unsuspected renal artery stenosis. J Vasc Surg 18(3):433-439

van der Velden J, van Bockel J, Zwartendijk J, van Krieken J, Terpstra JL (1992) Long-term results of surgical treatment of renal carcinoma in solitary kidneys by extracorporeal resection and autotransplantation. Br J Urol 69(5): 486-490

Vaziri ND, Barnes J, Khosrow M, Ehrlich R, Rosen SM (1976) Compression neuropathy subsequent to renal transplantation. Urology 7(2):145-147

CHAPTER 6

Renal Artery Atherosclerosis

Aksel Foss, Arnt Jakobsen, and Dagfinn Albrechtsen

6.1
Introduction

Atherosclerosis is the most common renal artery disease in adults, accounting for two thirds of all stenotic lesions (Fergany et al. 1995). Fibromuscular dysplasia accounts for the remaining third (Libertino and Beckmann 1994). Renal angiography often demonstrates uni- or bilateral atherosclerotic renal artery lesions, concurrent with atherosclerotic lesions of the abdominal aorta as well as vessels of other organ systems, especially of the coronary vessels (Dean et al. 1984; Novick et al. 1987; Tarazi et al. 1987; O'Mara et al. 1988; Allen et al. 1993). Atherosclerotic stenosis of the renal artery (RAS) characteristically involves the proximal segment of the artery extending from lesions of the aorta (Fig. 6.1). The left renal artery is most frequently affected, but bilateral lesions (Fig. 6.2) are seen in 30%-40% of patients (Libertino and Beckmann 1994). In the renal artery as in other arteries, atherosclerosis is more common in men than women. The mean age at the time of diagnosis is approximately 55 years. Estimates of the prevalence of atherosclerotic RAS vary from less than 1% to 10% (Ram 1992) of the hypertensive population. However, Scoble and colleagues (1989) observed a prevalence of atherosclerotic RAS as high as 14% in patients older than 50 years who were referred to a dialysis program.

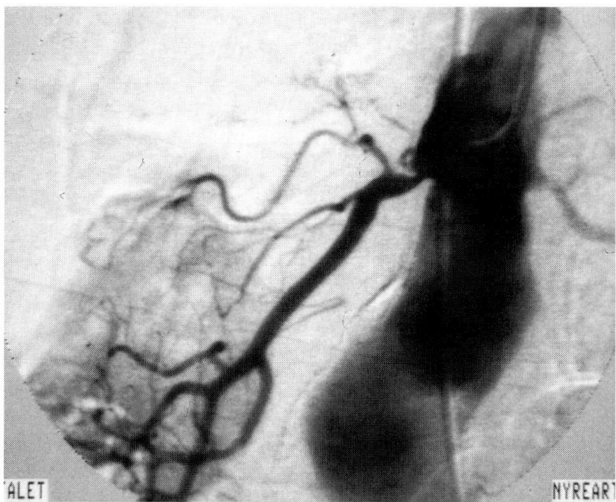

Fig. 6.1. Atherosclerotic RAS extending from atherosclerosis of the aorta

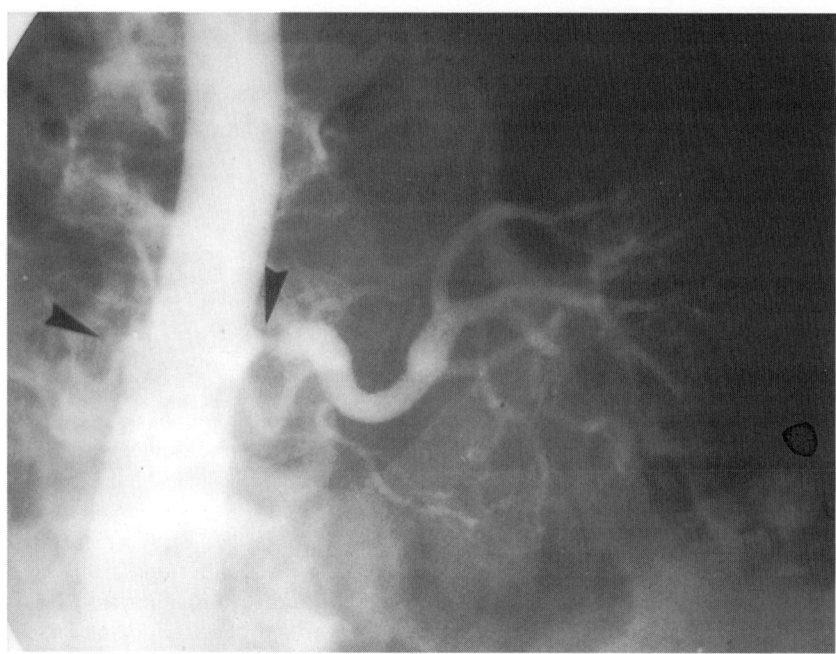

Fig. 6.2. Bilateral atherosclerotic renal artery lesions. A subtotal stenosis of the left renal artery and an occluded right artery

A morphological diagnosis of atherosclerotic RAS is not synonymous with atherosclerotic renovascular hypertension (RVH) (Dustan and de Wolfe 1964; Olin et al. 1990) and the prevalence of atherosclerotic RVH is therefore not precisely known (Sicard et al. 1995; see Chap. 1). The rate is influenced by age, sex, and race, as well as by the criteria used to define hypertension. With an aging population and an increasing prevalence of generalized atherosclerotic disease, more patients with bilateral severe atherosclerotic RAS associated with severe hypertension and renal dysfunction are being identified.

The difficulty in establishing a causal relationship between RAS and hypertension has led to the development of a variety of diagnostic tests to screen patients with hypertension for evidence of RVH and to evaluate the significance of an identified RAS (Ram 1992; see Chap. 1). A major drawback of such tests is that they rely on comparing a relatively normal kidney to one with RAS. In the clinical situation, however, there is often involvement of both renal arteries or there is renal parenchymal disease. Therefore, these tests often do not provide useful information (Sicard et al. 1995). Diagnostic tests for renal disease, such as intravenous pyelography, captopril renal scintigraphy, plasma renin levels, and selective renal vein renins, have shown to be insensitive and nonspecific in patients with bilateral disease (Lewis et al. 1976; Grim et al. 1979; Thornbury et al. 1982). Standard aorto-renal angiography is the most accepted technique for diagnosing atherosclerotic RAS. The clinical significance of renal artery disease can ultimately only be established by an improvement or cure of hypertension after correction of the demonstrated lesion.

In recent years, surgical revascularization is increasingly being used for the primary purpose of preserving renal function in patients with ischemic nephropathy caused by atherosclerotic RAS (Sos et al. 1983). Besides treatment of RVH, this is currently an important indication for surgical renal revascularization in patients with atherosclerotic RAS.

6.2
Atherosclerotic Renal Artery Senosis: The Natural Story

The natural development of atherosclerotic renal artery disease has been elucidated in several studies (Hunt and Strong 1973; Dean et al. 1981; Schreiber et al. 1984). Wollenweber et al. (1968) described the anatomical progression of atherosclerotic RAS in 30 patients by serial angiography. During a follow-up of 42 months, 12% of the initial nonazotemic patients developed end-stage renal failure. Another 20% of the patients had a significant impairment of kidney function. The 5-year survival rate of the study population was significantly lower, only being 72.6% of that of the expected survival rate for a comparable normal population. Half of the patients with severe atherosclerotic RAS, had definite atherosclerotic lesions in other organ systems. Schreiber et al. (1984), attempted to characterize the progression of the disease and to determine clinical markers of progression in 169 patients with atherosclerotic renal artery disease. Eighty-five of these patients were examined with two or more renal angiograms. Progression of the atherosclerotic lesions was observed in 40 patients and complete occlusion of the renal artery in 13 patients. Serum creatinine increased in half of the patients with progressive atherosclerotic disease, but only in 25% of the patients who were without evidence of angiographic progression. The size of the involved kidney decreased in 70% of the patients with progressive disease and in 25% of patients without progressive atherosclerotic disease. A decline in renal function and a decrease in kidney size were more common in patients with progressive atherosclerotic disease, compared to patients in whom the stenosis remained stable. Schreiber et al. (1984) conclude that serial serum creatinine measurements, in conjunction with measurements of kidney size, are useful markers of progressive atherosclerotic renovascular disease. A similar relationship between serum creatinine and reduced kidney size was not evident in individuals with RAS caused by fibromuscular dysplasia. The study clearly demonstrated that patients with high grade atherosclerotic RAS were at an increased risk of having clinically significant detoriation of renal function over time.

6.3
Management of Blood Pressure in Atherosclerotic RVH

Most cases of renovascular hypertension (RVH), can be managed medically with modern antihypertensive drugs (Hunt et al. 1974). However, medical treatment does not prevent progression of the atherosclerotic lesions and subsequent progressive renal failure. Hunt et al. (1974) reported a prospective study of 214 patients with RVH followed for 7-14 years. The overall survival rate was found to be significantly better for patients treated surgically as against patients treated medically (70% vs 38%

respectively), comparing both groups with the expected survival rate for a normal population. Dean et al. (1981) studied the impact of medical therapy of RVH on renal mass and function. Serial renal function studies were performed on 41 patients with RVH secondary to atherosclerotic renal artery disease and these authors concluded that progressive deterioration of renal function in medically treated patients with atherosclerotic RAS and RVH is common, and occurs even in the presence of adequate blood pressure management with drugs.

6.4
Percutanous Transluminal Renal Angioplasty vs Surgery

The role of surgery in the management of RAS has changed in recent years owing to the development of percutaneous transluminal renal angioplasty (PTA) (see Chap. 4). Maxwell et al. (1972) have established a set of criteria for treatment of RVH; cure is achieved if the diastolic blood pressure is reduced to 90 mmHg or less with at least 10 mmHg decrease from pretreatment level. Improvement is achieved if the diastolic blood pressure is reduced by 15% or more and diastolic blood pressure ranges between 90 and 110 mm Hg. Renal function is defined as improved if serum creatinine levels are reduced by more than 15% and as stable if the creatinine is unchanged or reduced by less than 15%. According to these criteria, several large studies on PTA in patients with RAS have reported cure rates of 15%-25% and improved rates of approximately 45%-60% after 36-60 months follow-up, regarding hypertension and renal function (Sos et al. 1983; Martin et al. 1985; Baert et al. 1990; Martin et al. 1992). The effect of PTA in the treatment of elevated blood pressure due to RAS caused by fibromuscular dysplasia has been shown to be excellent. PTA is now the treatment of choice in fibromuscular dysplasia. Atherosclerotic lesions on the other hand, especially those involving the ostium and the wall of the aorta are often said to be more resistant to standard PTA. Several studies have reported that 20%-40% of patients with atherosclerotic renovascular disease do not benefit from PTA (Cicuto et al. 1981; Council on Scientific Affairs 1984; Brawn and Ramsay 1987). In contrast to these results, Weibull et al. (1993) performed a prospective study of 58 patients with unilateral atherosclerotic RAS randomized to either PTA or surgical treatment. Successful treatment was defined as total elimination of the stenosis. Angiography was performed 10 days, 1 year, and 2 years after treatment to verify patency. Blood pressure and renal function were simultaneously evaluated. The patency rate after 24 months was 75% in the PTA group and 96% in the surgical group. Hypertension was cured or improved in 83% of the PTA treated patients and in 89% of the surgically treated patients. Renal function was improved or stable in 96% of the PTA group and 75% of the surgical group. They conclude that PTA is recommended as first choice of therapy for atherosclerotic RAS, causing RVH if combined with intensive follow-up and aggressive reintervention.

Atherosclerotic disease involving the branches of the renal artery may be difficult to recognize because of sparse symptoms. These complex renal artery lesions are often inaccessible to PTA, but can successfully be treated by ex vivo microsurgical reconstruction (Harris et al. 1991).

Rupture of the artery, occlusion, and postinterventional pseudoaneurysms are well known complications of PTA. These complications can cause irretrievable injury to the patient, particularly when treating stenosis on a solitary functioning kidney. Experienced surgical backup is therefore necessary when PTA is used to treat RAS.

In summary, PTA is the treatment of choice in patients with renal artery lesions causing hypertension or renal failure and when there are contraindications to surgical treatment. Improved results could perhaps be achieved by recent technological advances, such as intraluminal artery stents to prevent elastic recoil and stenosis. Surgical backup is essential when performing PTA.

6.5
Surgical Management of Atherosclerotic Renal Disease

Interest in surgical treatment of lesions of the renal arteries has varied considerably over the last 30 years. Various surgical methods have been used, e.g., local endarterectomy and bypass surgery from the aorta using homologous vein, artery, or prosthetic grafts (Davis et al. 1979; Ying et al. 1984; Novick et al. 1987; Scoble et al. 1989). If the aorta is severely affected by atherosclerotic disease or has previously undergone surgery, extra-anatomic bypasses from miscellaneous arteries, such as the hepatic, gastroduodenal, splenic, and mesenteric arteries have been performed (Novick et al. 1987; Sicard et al. 1995). There have been few published studies on the results of autotransplantation in the treatment of RVH. Most authors recommend an in situ bypass operation for central atherosclerotic stenosis of the renal artery (Maxwell et al. 1972; Chibaro et al. 1984; Moncure et al. 1986; Messina et al. 1992; Libertino and Beckman 1994; Novick 1994; Reilly et al. 1994). Furthermore most publications on autotransplantation with ex vivo renal artery repair report patients with fibromuscular dysplasia or peripheral RAS (Dubernard et al. 1985a; Jordan et al. 1985; Van Bockel et al. 1988; Barral et al. 1992; Brekke et al. 1992). The studies are often hampered by heterogeneous patient groups and poor definitions regarding RVH and renal function. Dubernard et al. (1985b) reported that autotransplantation with ex vivo reconstruction of the renal vessels was superior to in situ bypass techniques in the surgical treatment of RVH caused by lesions which extended into the branches of the renal artery. They claim that autotransplantation represents a better alternative in the surgical treatment of this condition. Kaufmann et al. (1979) have shown in 266 bypass procedures for RVH that 67% of the patients were cured while 20% of the patients showed improvements. Hypertension is, however, not defined in the paper. They also performed 59 autotransplantations with extracorporeal renal artery repair, curing and improving renovascular hypertension in 88% and 5% of the cases, respectively. Novick et al. (1987) performed 254 operations in 241 patients with renal artery disease caused by atherosclerosis. Of these, 232 were bypass operations and 8 autotransplantations. One hundred and eighty patients were operated on for hypertension, defined as blood pressure >140/90, and 161 patients underwent surgery to preserve renal function or for renal failure and RVH combined. Impaired renal function was defined as serum creatinine 20% above normal. Hypertension was cured in 30.6% and improved in 61.1% of the patients. Renal function improved in 58%, remained stable in 31.1%, and detoriated in 11.2% of the patients.

6.6
Renal Autotransplantation in Atherosclerotic Renal Disease

We have used our experience from our living donor kidney transplant program, which started in 1969, to offer the service of renal autotransplantation for patients having RVH and/or ischemic nephropathy caused by atherosclerotic stenosis in the periostial region of the renal artery (see Chap. 7). Since 1973, 140 autotransplantations have been performed in 122 patients suffering from RVH caused by periostial stenotic atherosclerotic lesions in the renal artery. All patients had hypertension >140/90 despite antihypertensive therapy (1-4 drugs). Twenty-seven patients (22%) had bilateral lesions. Eight patients (7%) had bilateral autotransplantation performed in the same session. Twenty-one patients (17%) had only one functioning kidney, and one patient had bilateral renal artery occlusion and was operated with simultaneous autotransplantation of both kidneys. The remaining 74 patients had unilateral lesions at angiography. Only 43% of the patients had normal kidney function (serum creatinine <130 µmol/l). Thirty-one patients (25%) had serum creatinines of 131-199 µmol/l, another 30 patients had levels between 200-499, and nine patients (7%) had levels above 500 µmol (550 to 800 µmol/l) (Table 6.1). Eighty-two patients were men. The mean age was 56.1 years (range 37-75). Ten patients were below 40 years of age, 27 between 40 and 49 years, 37 between 50 and 59 years, and 48 patients (33%) were more than 60 years of age. Seven patients were more than 70 years of age. The follow-up time ranged from 6 months to 10 years (Table 6.2). The technique for autotransplantation is described elsewhere (see Chap. 5). The operation time averaged 7.9 h, ranging from 4.75 h to 11.5 h. All procedures were technically successful. The early postoperative mortality (<30 days) was 7% (eight patients), with a mean age of 66.7 years. Four patients died of coronary infarction, one patient of cerebral hemorrhage, and three patients of septicemia and multiorgan failure. Functional loss of the autograft in the follow up time occurred in 20 patients (16%). Ten of these patients had preoperative renal malfunction with serum creatinine levels from 163 to 800 µmol/l. Two of the lost autografts were retrospectively judged to be nonfunctioning preoperatively [effective renal plasma flow (ERPF) 15 and 20 ml/min respectively]. Another six patients had functional loss of the autotransplant due to stenosis or thrombosis of the transplant artery 4 months to 3 years (mean 17 months) following the operation The other four patients lost their grafts for various reasons, one because of sepsis in the early postoperative phase, one at 6 months because of an undiagnosed ureteral obstruction, and one at 1 year due to possible irradiation damage following treatment for cancer of the cervix uteri. One kidney loss occurred at 18 months for an undefined reason.

Table 6.1. Preoperative serum creatinine levels in 122 patients treated surgically with vascular reconstruction and autotransplantation for atherosclerotic RAS

No. of patients (%)	Serum creatinine (µmol/l)
52 (43%)	<130
31 (25%)	131–199
30 (25%)	200–499
9 (7%)	500–800

Table 6.2. Age, gender and follow-up in 122 patients treated surgically with vascular reconstruction and autotransplantation for atherosclerotic RAS

Population			
Men	Women	Age	Follow-up (in years)
82	40	56.1 (37-75)	0.5-10

Twenty-one percent of the patients normalized their blood pressure without medication. Another 60% improved their blood pressure significantly, resulting in a reduced requirement for antihypertensive drugs (Table 6.3). Of 21 patients having autotransplantation of a single functioning kidney, 18 patients (86%) retained autograft function during the follow-up period. Serum creatinine in these patients improved from an average of 242 μmol/l to 189 μmol/l. In total, renal function improved or was unchanged in 87%. Improvement was defined as a decrease in serum creatinine by more than 20%. Deterioriation of renal function was seen in 13% of the patients.

Table 6.3. Effect on blood pressure and serum creatinine 3-6 months following vascular reconstruction and autotransplantation in 122 patients treated for atherosclerotic RAS

	Normalized (%)	Improved (%)	Unchanged (%)	Deteriorated (%)
Blood pressure	21	60	19	0
Creatinine		20	67	13

Our therapeutic management of patients with atherosclerotic RAS in the periostial region has somewhat changed since the introduction of renal PTA by Gruntzig and collaborators in 1978. The primary procedure is now PTA, using metallic stents if required. If this does not succeed in improving hypertension and/or stabilizing or improving renal function, we find autotransplantation with ex vivo arterial repair to be indicated. Furthermore, autotransplantation is also recommended for patients with an occluded renal artery, provided adequate renal perfusion and renal mass have been preserved by extrarenal circulation, as evidenced by renal angiography, renal scintigraphy, and CT scans.

6.7
Summary

Aorto-renal bypass surgery is generally considered to be a safe and effective treatment for RAS. The technique, however, is not universally applicable to all kinds of stenoses and therefore burdened with several weaknesses. Surgical exposure is difficult. The surgeon has to master vascular surgery deep in the renal fossa. Cold perfusion of the in situ kidney is complicated, especially when treating branch renal artery lesions.

Autotransplantation with ex vivo repair allows optimal exposure for a microvascular technique in a bloodless field, with controlled hypothermic protection of the kidney.

PTA has been shown to be an excellent treatment for patients with fibromuscular dysplasia. It is also our first choice of treatment for patients with atherosclerotic RAS. But for patients inadequately treated with PTA and for patients with renal artery occlusion, with preserved renal parenchyma, we suggest autotransplantation with ex vivo renal artery repair as the treatment of choice. It is safe, preservation of renal function is good, and the effect on blood pressure is excellent. However, it should be kept in mind that atherosclerotic renal artery disease is primarily a condition of the elderly. In our material, one third of the patients were over 60. Atherosclerotic RAS is frequently combined with atherosclerotic lesions in other arteries, especially the coronary arteries. A preoperative cardiac evaluation is therefore necessary, including a coronary angiography and, when indicated, a coronary bypass prior to autotransplantation. The postoperative deaths in our series were mainly caused by myocardial infarction; we now perform coronary angiography on all patients over 40 with atherosclerotic renal artery stenoses.

Our results indicate that the efficacy of autotransplantation in treating hypertension and preserving renal function is equally good or better than bypass techniques. However, a successful program for autotransplantation with ex vivo renal artery repair depends on training and experience in living donor nephrectomy and kidney transplantation. The kidney should be harvested, using an atraumatic technique for optimal kidney preservation. The surgeon should be trained in hypothermic protection of the transplant. He or she should be familiar with microvascular surgery and the technique for transplanting the kidney to the iliac vessels, including reimplantation of the ureter into the bladder.

References

Allen BT, Rubin BG, Anderson CB, Thompson RW, Sicard GA (1993) Simultaneous surgical management of aortic and renovascular disease. Am J Surg 166(6):726-732

Baert AL, Wilms G, Amery A, Vermylen J, Suy R (1990) Percutaneous transluminal renal angioplasty: initial results and long-term follow-up in 202 patients. Cardiovasc Intervent Radiol 13(1):22-28

Barral X, Gournier JP, Frering V, Favre JP, Berthoux F (1992) Dysplastic lesions of renal artery branches: late results of ex vivo repair. Ann Vasc Surg 6(3):225-231

Brawn LA, Ramsay LE (1987) Is "improvement" real with percutaneous transluminal angioplasty in the management of RVH? Lancet 2(8571):1313-1316

Brekke IB, Sødal G, Jakobsen A, Bentdal O, Pfeffer P, Albrechtsen D, Flatmark A (1992) Fibro-muscular renal artery disease treated by extracorporeal vascular reconstruction and renal autotransplantation: short- and long-term results. Eur J Vasc Surg 6(5):471-476

Chibaro EA, Libertino JA, Novick AC (1984) Use of the hepatic circulation for renal revascularization. Ann Surg 199(4):406-411

Cicuto KP, McLean GK, Oleaga JA, Freiman DB, Grossman RA, Ring EJ (1981) RAS: anatomic classification for percutaneous transluminal angioplasty. AJR 137(3):599-601

Council on Scientific Affairs (1984) Percutaneous transluminal angioplasty. JAMA 251:764-768

Davis BA, Crook JE, Vestal RE, Oates JA (1979) Prevalence of renovascular hypertension in patients with grade III or IV hypertensive retinopathy. N Engl J Med 301:1273-1276

Dean RH, Kieffer RW, Smith BM, Oates JA, Nadeau JH, Hollifield JW, DuPont WD (1981) RVH: anatomic and renal function changes during drug therapy. Arch Surg 116(11):1408-1415

Dean RH, Keyser JE, DuPont WD, Nadeau JH, Meacham PW (1984) Aortic and renal vascular disease. Factors affecting the value of combined procedures. Ann Surg 200(3):336-344

Dubernard JM, Martin X, Gelet A, Mongin D, Canton F, Tabib A (1985a) Renal autotransplantation versus bypass techniques for RVH. Surgery 97(5):529-534

Dubernard JM, Martin X, Mongin D, Gelet A, Canton F (1985b) Extracorporeal replacement of the renal artery: techniques, indications and long-term results. J Urol 133(1):13-16

Dustan HP, de Wolfe VG (1964) Normal artery pressure in patients with renal artery stenosis. JAMA 187:1028-1029

Fergany AMR, Kolettis P, Novick C (1995) The contemporary role of extra-anatomical surgical renal revascularization in patients with atherosclerotic renal artery disease. J Urol 153:1798-1802

Grim CE, Luft FC, Weinberger MH, Grim CM (1979) Sensitivity and specificity of screening tests for renal vascular hypertension. Ann Intern Med 91:617-622

Gruntzig A, Kuhlman U, Vetter W, Lutolf U, Meier B, Siegenthaler W (1978) Treatment of RVH with percutaneous transluminal dilatation of a renal-artery stenosis. Lancet 1:801-802

Harris JP, Walker PJ, White GH, May J (1991) Bench repair of complex renal arterial lesions. Ann Vasc Surg 5(2):138-142

Hunt JC, Strong CG (1973) RVH. Mechanisms, natural history and treatment. Am J Cardiol 32(4):562-574

Hunt JC, Sheps SG, Harrison EG Jr., Strong CG, Bernatz PE (1974) Renal and RVH. A reasoned approach to diagnosis and management. Arch Intern Med 133(6):988-999

Jordan ML, Novick AC, Cunningham RL (1985) The role of renal autotransplantation in pediatric and young adult patients with renal artery disease. J Vasc Surg 2(3):385-392

Kaufman JJ (1979) RVH: the UCLA experience (review). J Urol 121(2):139-144

Lewis PF, Bulpitt CH, Sherwood T, Dollery CT (1976) Routine intravenous urography in the investigation of hypertension. J Chron Dis 29:785-792

Libertino JA, Beckmann CF (1994) Surgery and percutaneous angioplasty in the management of RVH (review). Urol Clin North Am 21(2):235-243

Martin LG, Cork RD, Kaufman SL (1992) Long-term results of angioplasty in 110 patients with RAS. J Vasc Interv Radiol 3(4):619-626

Martin LG, Price RB, Casarella WJ, Sones PJ, Wells JO Jr, Zellmer RA, Chuang VP, Silbiger ML Jr, Berkman WA (1985) Percutaneous angioplasty in clinical management of RVH: initial and long-term results. Radiology 155(3):629-633

Maxwell MH, Bleifer KH, Franklin SS, Varady PD (1972) Cooperative study of RVH. Demographic analysis of the study. JAMA 220(9):1195-1204

Messina LM, Zelenock GB, Yao KA, Stanley JC (1992) Renal revascularization for recurrent pulmonary edema in patients with poorly controlled hypertension and renal insufficiency: a distinct subgroup of patients with arteriosclerotic renal artery occlusive disease. J Vasc Surg 15(1):73-80

Moncure AC, Brewster DC, Darling RC, Atnip RG, Newton WD, Abbott WM (1986) Use of the splenic and hepatic arteries for renal revascularization. J Vasc Surg 3(2):196-203

Novick AC, Ziegelbaum M, Vidt DG, Gifford RW Jr, Pohl MA, Goormastic M (1987) Trends in surgical revascularization for renal artery disease. Ten years' experience. JAMA 257(4):498-501

Novick AC (1994) Atherosclerotic ischemic nephropathy. Epidemiology and clinical considerations (review). Urol Clin North Am 21(2):195-200

Olin JW, Melia M, Young JR, Graor RA, Risius B (1990) Prevalence of atherosclerotic RAS in patients with atherosclerosis elsewhere. Am J Med 88(1N):46N-51N

O'Mara CS, Maples MD, Kilgore TL Jr, McMullan MH, Tyler HB, Mundinger GH Jr, Kennedy RE (1988) Simultaneous aortic reconstruction and bilateral renal revascularization. Is this a safe and effective procedure? (See comments) J Vasc Surg 8(4):357-366

Ram CV (1992) Current concepts in RVH (review). Am J Med Sci 304(1):53-71

Reilly JM, Rubin BG, Thompson RW, Allen BT, Anderson CB, Sicard GA (1994) Long-term effectiveness of extraanatomic renal artery revascularization. Surgery 116(4):784-790

Schreiber MJ, Pohl MA, Novick AC (1984) The natural history of atherosclerotic and fibrous renal artery disease. Urol Clin North Am 11(3):383-392

Scoble JE, Maher ER, Hamilton G, Dick R, Sweny P, Moorhead JF (1989) Atherosclerotic renovascular disease causing renal impairment - a case for treatment. Clin Nephrol 31(3):119-122

Sicard GA, Reilly JM, Picus DD, Allen BT (1995) Alternatives in renal revascularization (review). Curr Probl Surg 32(7):571-652

Sos TA, Pickering TG, Sniderman K, Saddekni S, Case DB, Silane MF, Vaughan ED Jr, Laragh JH (1983) Percutaneous transluminal renal angioplasty in renovascular hypertension due to atheroma or fibromuscular dysplasia. N Engl J Med 309(5):274-279

Tarazi RY, Hertzer NR, Beven EG, O'Hara PJ, Anton GE, Krajewski LP (1987) Simultaneous aortic reconstruction and renal revascularization: risk factors and late results in eighty-nine patients. J Vasc Surg 5(5):707-714

Thornbury JR, Stanley JC, Fryback DG (1982) Hypertensive urogram: a non-discrimatory test for RVH. AJR 138:43-49

Van Bockel JH, van Schilfgaarde R, Overbosch EH, Felthuis W, Terpstra JL (1988) The influence of the surgical technique upon the short term and long term anatomic results in reconstructive operation for RVH. Surg Gynecol Obstet 166(5):402-408

Weibull H, Bergqvist D, Bergentz SE, Jonsson K, Hulthen L, Manhem P (1993) Percutaneous transluminal renal angioplasty versus surgical reconstruction of atherosclerotic RAS: a prospective randomized study. J Vasc Surg 18(5):841-850

Wollenweber J, Sheps SG, Davis GD (1968) Clinical course of atherosclerotic renovascular disease. Am J Cardiol 21(1):60-71

Ying CY, Tifft CP, Garvas H, Chobavian AV (1984) Renal revascularization in the azotemic hypertensive patient resistant to therapy. N Eng J Med 311:1070-1075

The Role of Bench Surgery in the Treatment of Renal Artery Stenoses and Aneurysms Caused by Fibromuscular Dysplasia

Inge B. Brekke and Bjørn Lien

7.1
Introduction

The term fibromuscular dysplasia (FMD) encompasses an entity of nonatherosclerotic, noninflammatory segmental angiopathies that usually involve medium- and small-sized arteries. A classification has been developed based on the arterial layer (intima, media, or adventitia) in which the lesions predominate (Harrison and McCormack 1971; Stanley et al. 1975). The most common form, medial fibroplasia, is characterized by multifocal stenoses caused by fibromuscular proliferation forming ridges replacing the normal intimal and medial structure. This may alternate with areas of mural thinning and dilation, giving the characteristic "string of beads" arteriographic appearance (Fig. 7.1). Solitary stenoses (Fig. 7.2A) caused by intimal, medial, perimedial, or adventitial hyperplasia, or aneurysms in dysplastic mural lesions (Fig. 7.2C) are also frequently observed.

First described in the renal artery in 1938 (Leadbetter and Burkland 1938), FMD is most commonly observed in the renal, carotid, and intracerebral arteries, but has also

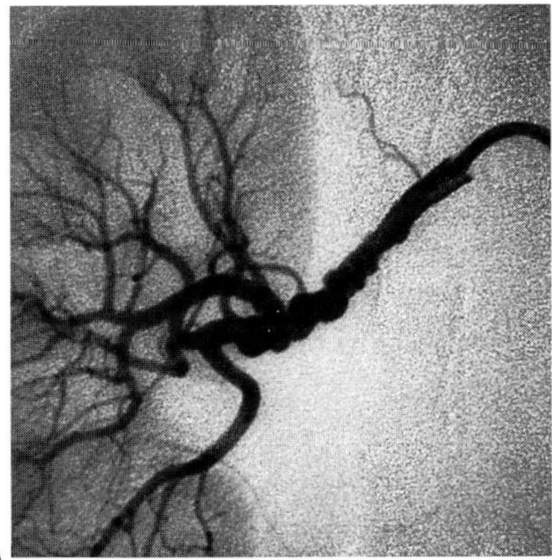

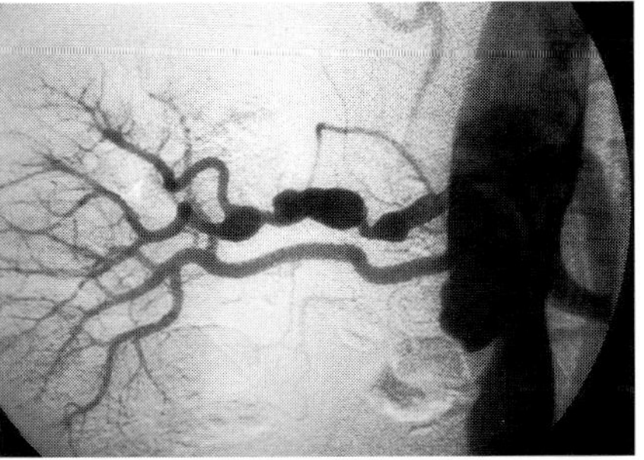

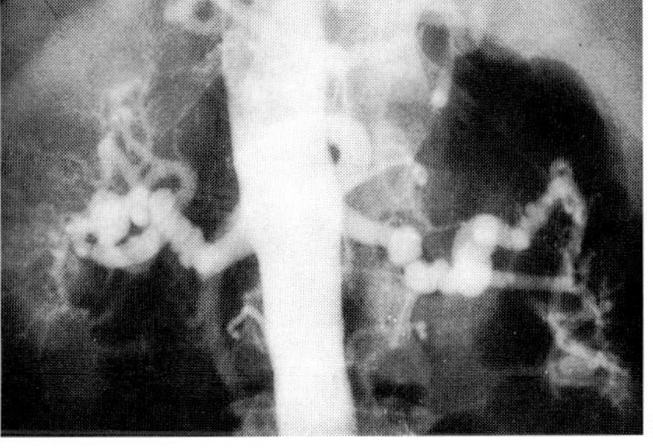

Fig. 7.1 A–C. Typical „string of beads" appearance of renal artery (A). Multiple stenoses and microaneurysms in one of two renal arteries (B). Bilateral renal artery fibromuscular dysplasia (C)

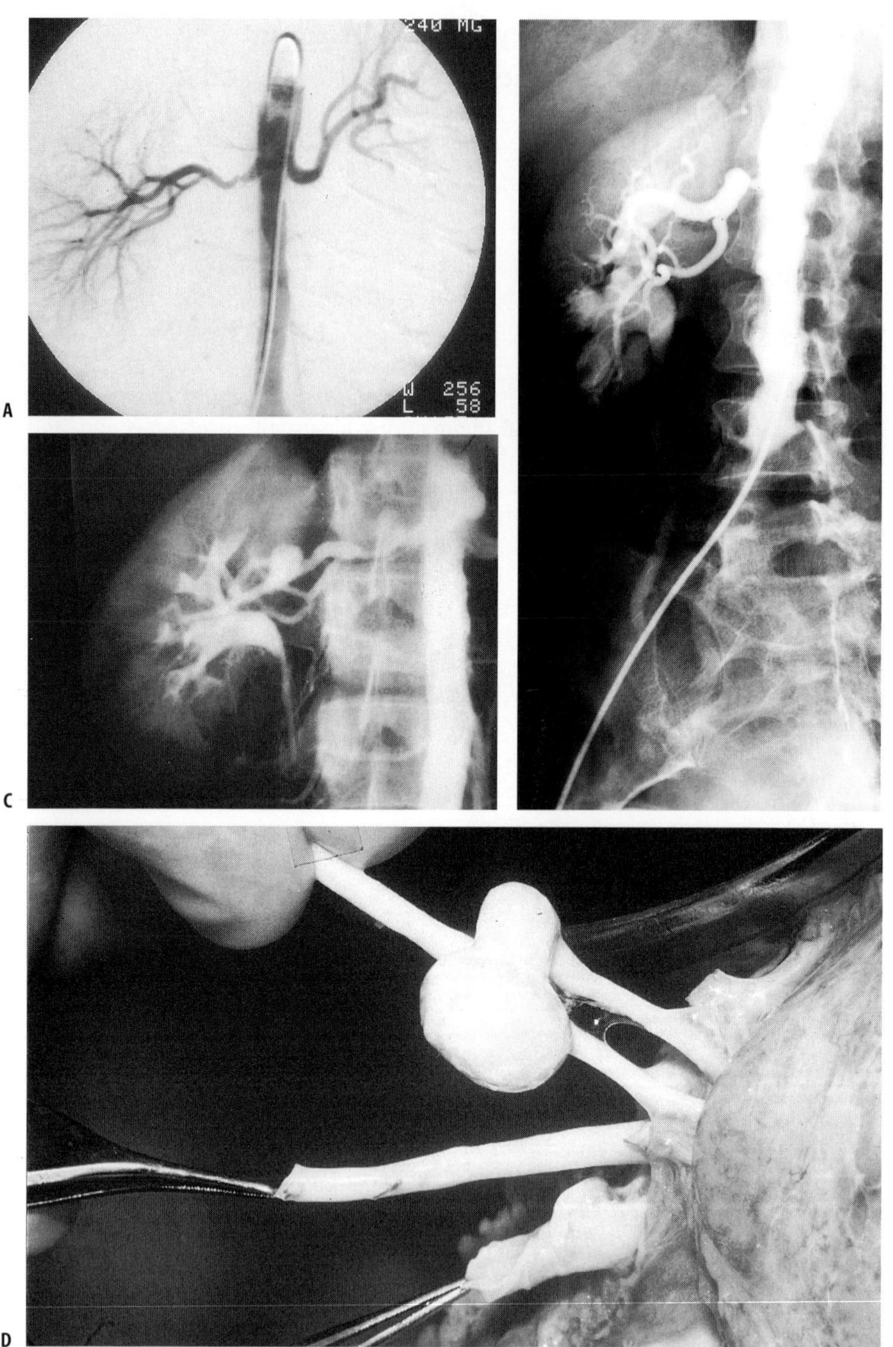

Fig. 7.2 A–D. Solitary renal artery stenosis caused by FMD (A), and atherosclerosis (B). Typical renal artery aneurysm caused by FMD, as seen on the angiogram (C) and ex vivo (D)

been described in the brachial, femoral, coronary, visceral, iliac, and other arteries (Lüscher et al. 1987; Lin et al. 1992; Ritota et al. 1994; Ertel et al.1994), and probably may be found in any arterial tree.

This vascular disease of unknown etiology occurs in all age groups, predominantly in females (Ekelund et al. 1978; George et al. 1989). Familial occurrence has occasionally been described (Simon et al. 1972), and casuistics of the angiopathy associated with various generalized connective tissue disorders have been published (Schievink et al. 1994).

Autopsy studies have demonstrated a prevalence of renal artery FMD of 1%–2% of the general population (Heffelfinger et al. 1970). Next to atherosclerotic lesions, FMD is the most common cause of renovascular hypertension (RVH) in adults, and RVH in children is claimed to be caused by FMD in up to 95% of all cases (Stanley 1984; Dillon 1994).The right kidney is more frequently affected than the left, but bilateral renal implication (Fig. 7.1C) is diagnosed in 30%–70% of the cases (Maxwell et al. 1972; Ekelund et al. 1978). Solitary or multifocal stenoses of the main renal artery or branches are the most common features of renal FMD, but FMD is also the most common cause of renal artery aneurysms (Dzsinich et al. 1993; Brekke et al. 1992).

In our published series of 237 patients undergoing surgery for renal artery pathology, FMD was diagnosed in 59 (25%), with a mean patient age of 35 years (range 2–66). Forty-one (69%) of these were females. Eleven patients were younger than 16 years of age. In 21 patients (36%), FMD was bilateral at the time of surgery or developed in the contralateral kidney during follow-up. A renal artery aneurysm was the indication for surgery in 21 (33%) of the 63 kidneys treated (Brekke et al. 1992).

7.2
Diagnosis

Both stenotic and aneurysmal renal artery disease are often associated with hypertension, which leads to diagnostic intervention. A secondary cause of hypertension should be suspected in patients with malignant hypertension and in hypertension refractory to what would seem appropriate medical therapy, especially when the onset is in patients younger than 30 or older than 50 years of age. In children, FMD is the most common cause of RVH, and arteriography is recommended for all patients in whom a nonvascular cause for the hypertension has not been established.

Ideally, the diagnosis of RVH requires not only the demonstration of renal artery pathology, but also evidence of renal ischemia, the cardinal functional component in RVH. However, the sensitivity and specificity of methods for screening and diagnosing RVH, such as intravenous pyelography, renal vein renin determination, and captopril renography (see Chaps. 1–3), have been disappointing and we have stopped the routine use of these tests. When renal artery FMD is angiographically diagnosed in a hypertensive patient, there is usually no doubt that the anatomical lesion is the cause of the hypertension, and further diagnostic examination is normally unnecessary. Visual identification of the anatomical details of the renal vasculature is fundamental for interventional therapy, and renal arteriography is therefore essential for the evaluation of these conditions (see Chap. 2). While atherosclerosis characteristically involves the proximal portion of the renal artery (Fig. 7.2B), FMD is usually located in the distal part or in branches of the renal artery, causing stenosis or aneurysm formation (Figs. 7.1, 7.2A,C).

In our series of 63 kidneys treated with bench surgery for renal artery FMD, the diagnosis was based on characteristic angiographical appearance and was histologically confirmed postoperatively.

7.3
Indications for Surgery

Hypertension and stenoses threatening kidney function are the most common indications for intervention, as in 95% of the patients in our series (Brekke et al. 1992). Renal artery FMD lesions progress over time, and intervention should be undertaken to prevent complete artery occlusion. Resection of a renal artery aneurysm may also occasionally be indicated for local symptoms or to obviate the risk of aneurysm rupture. The hypertension often associated with aneurysms is probably secondary to the renal ischemia caused by turbulent flow.

Advances in the surgical management of RVH have evolved over the past decades such that carefully performed reconstruction benefits 85%–95% of properly selected patients (Stanley 1994). However, the role of surgery in the management of renal artery stenoses has changed in recent years due to the development of percutaneous transluminal angioplasty (PTA). PTA has superseded surgery in most institutions as the first line of treatment for most stenotic lesions involving the renal vasculature. The results of PTA in the treatment of FMD with stenosis of the main renal artery are admirable (Klinge et al. 1989; Tegtmeyer et al. 1991). PTA is, therefore, now the treatment of choice in these cases. A recent series has also documented excellent technical success rates in branch involvement (Cluzel et al. 1994). However, PTA has its limitations and is not without complications as previously reported (Dean et al. 1987; Klinge et al.1989; Tegtmeyer et al. 1991). In our own series of 27 kidneys autotransplanted for total renal artery occlusion, five of the occlusions occurred during PTA attempts. To avoid serious complications it has been advocated to limit the routine use of PTA to nonorificial stenoses of the main renal artery in patients with two functioning kidneys (Dean et al. 1987; Shifrin et al. 1991; Novick 1991). Surgery is indicated when aneurysms and complex branch renal artery stenoses preclude the use of PTA or when PTA has failed.

7.3.1
Hypertension

Selection of hypertensive patients for elective intervention may imply documentation that a renal artery lesion is of functional importance. However, as already mentioned, identification of patients that will benefit from correction of renal artery pathology has remained an elusive goal, and intervention must be based on the anatomy as seen on the angiogram.

The indication for surgery in patients with hypertension secondary to renal artery FMD is usually more liberal than in patients with atherosclerosis. The majority of patients are below 40–45 years of age and hypertension is often severe. Surgery should therefore, as a rule, be advocated in lesions not accessible by PTA.

7.3.2
Preservation and Restoration of Renal Function

FMD is usually a progressive disease, at least in persons less than 40–50 years of age, and the progress of FMD may lead to renal artery occlusion or aneurysm rupture when left untreated. Thus, to preserve renal function, prophylactic renal artery reconstruction is advisable in selected patients. Unilateral renal artery occlusion may be clinically silent, and the diagnosis is therefore often delayed. However, restoration of renal function, even after weeks of artery occlusion, has been shown to be conceivable (Perona et al. 1989), provided some renal circulation is maintained through capsular vessels (Fig. 7.3). Return of function may be expected if signs of collateral circulation can be angiographically demonstrated, if the distal renal artery is patent at the time of surgery, and if preserved glomerular structure is bioptically verified.

The true prevalence of renal artery aneurysms in the general population is not known. Aneurysms were identified in 1% of 8525 angiograms (Tham et al. 1983), whereas other studies have found a much lower incidence (Hageman et al. 1978), discrepancies that are probably due to variations in diagnostic accuracy. Improvements in imaging techniques have resulted in increased detection of this abnormality, but its management is still controversial. Potential aneurysm complications such as renal artery thrombosis or distal embolization appear to be rare. Aneurysm rupture, the most dramatic complication, is also rare, especially in the normotensive patient with a circumferentially calcified aneurysm (Harrow and Sloane 1959). In noncalcified or incompletely calcified aneurysms, rupture rates of 20%–30% have been published (Harrow and Sloane 1959; Ippolito and LeVeen 1960; Cerny et al. 1968). The increased

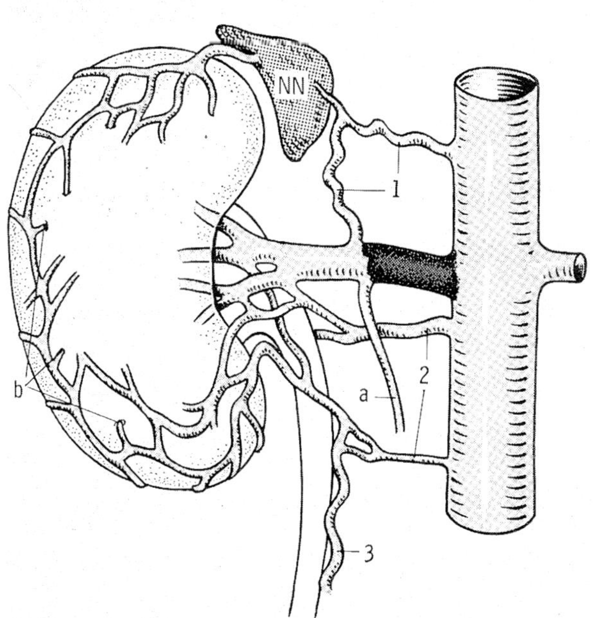

Fig. 7.3. Extrarenal collateral circulation following occlusion of the renal artery. Suprarenal artery (*1*). Lumbar arteries (*2*). Ureteral vascular system (*3*). Gonadal artery (*a*). Capsular arteries (*b*) (From Hallwachs and Vollmar 1971)

risk of rupture during pregnancy is probably due to hormonally induced changes in the aneurysm wall. The poor prognosis in this setting has prompted authors to recommend that a renal artery aneurysm of any size should be repaired prophylactically in women who may become pregnant (Cohen and Shamash 1987). Otherwise, the presence of hypertension, enlargement of the aneurysm, a solitary kidney, bilateral involvement, acute hematuria, or an aneurysm diameter of more than 1.5 cm are suggested indications for surgical treatment, especially in cases of noncalcified aneurysms (Poutasse 1975; Novick 1991; Dzsinich et al. 1993).

7.3.3
Loin Pain/Hematuria Syndrome

The loin pain/hematuria syndrome is a rare condition, predominantly affecting young women. Recurrent episodes of loin pain are associated with gross or microscopic hematuria (Little et al. 1967). Cases reported have been associated with aneurysmal or stenotic FMD of the renal artery, and renal autotransplantation has been demonstrated to effectively cure this syndrome (Sheil et al. 1985; Bloom et al. 1989; Brekke et al. 1992).

7.4
Choice of Surgical Technique

The surgeon's personal preferences and experience will be of importance when deciding on the type of surgery. However, several authors with extensive experience in both ex vivo and in situ renal artery repair have expressed their preference for ex vivo surgery, especially in the more complex abnormalities (Dubernard et al. 1985; Kent et al. 1987; van Bockel et al. 1989). The major advantages of the ex vivo technique over in situ revascularization methods are the excellent exposure of the renal artery branches and the exceptional fine working conditions provided by this approach. Thus, when second- and third-order branches are involved, particularly when aneurysmal disease involves multiple vessels, extracorporeal repair is the procedure of choice.

Belzer, one of the pioneers of bench surgery, gave the following indications for ex vivo renal artery repair (Belzer and Raczkowski 1982), most of which are still valid:

- Failure of medical antihypertensive treatment or deteriorating renal function
- Lesion not repairable by standard surgical techniques
- Bilateral disease or a solitary kidney
- Unilateral disease in young patients
- Failure of previous in situ reconstruction
- Aorta of very poor quality, but with no obstruction
- Unusual conditions, such as a renal artery aneurysm
- More than two vessels involved

7.5
Extracorporeal Renal Artery Reconstruction

When performing unilateral autotransplantation, the affected kidney is usually removed through a flank incision. The kidney is then perfused with chilled (4°C) Euro-Collins, Ringer's acetate, or other preservation solutions until the venous effluent is clear. While submerged in a basin with ice slush saline solution, the renal artery and its branches are carefully dissected distally as far as is required to reach normal artery beyond the diseased area. The affected portion of the artery is excised, and reconstruction may be performed by a variety of techniques. In most cases arterial reconstruction can be accomplished by variations of the „double barrel" technique alone (see Fig. 5.1), or in combination with the interposition of an autologous vein or artery graft as exemplified in Figs. 7.4A, 7.5 and 7.6B. Even though saphenous vein has been widely used to replace portions of the renal artery, the long-term effect of arterial blood flow on vein grafts has caused some concern about their use for this purpose, especially in younger patients. Therefore, most authors express a preference for arterial autografts. The internal iliac artery with its branches appears to be ideal for replacing parts of the renal arterial tree (Fig. 7.6). On the very rare occasion when neither an arterial nor a venous graft is available, a synthetic artery graft can be used, preferably a soft and easily sutured tetrafluoroethylene (Gor-Tex) graft. Excision of a short arterial segment and approximation of the cut ends by direct end-to-end anastomosis (Fig. 7.4B) or simple excision of the affected portion of the main renal artery (Fig. 7.4C) is possible when a very small portion of the artery is affected. Microvascular equipment, including 7/0–9/0 suture material, microsurgical instruments, and magnifying glasses, is used for all surgery on renal artery branches. Finally, when the reconstruction is completed, the arterial tree as well as the renal vein may be tested for leakage before autotransplantation.

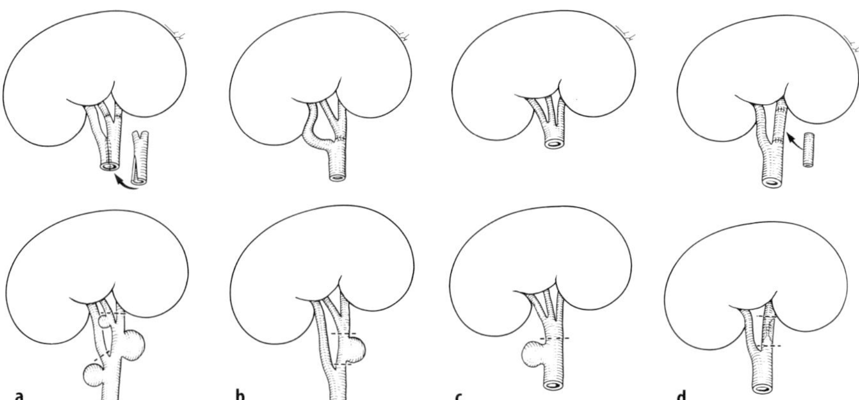

Fig. 7.4. Various methods applied for renal artery reconstruction

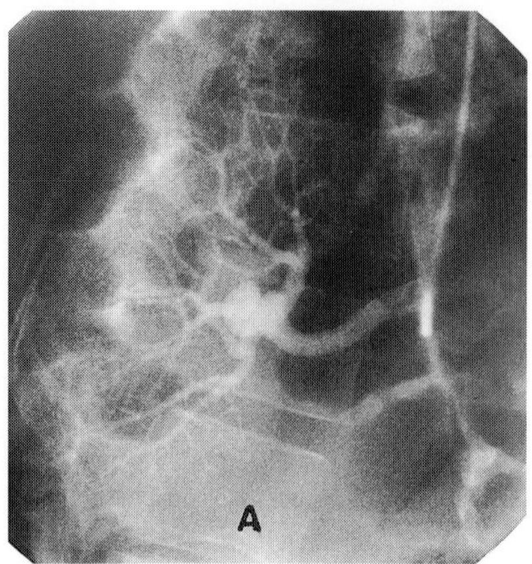

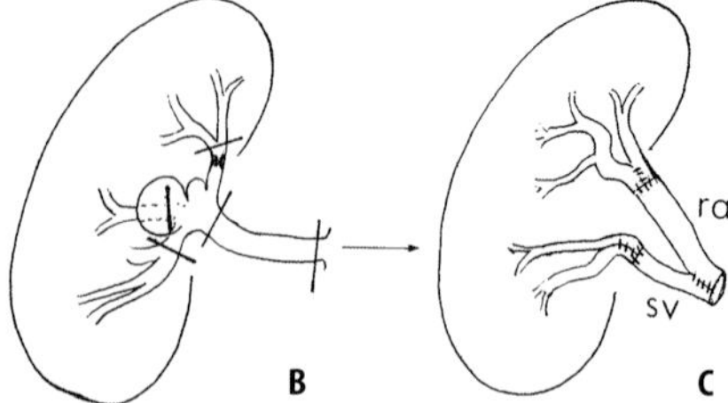

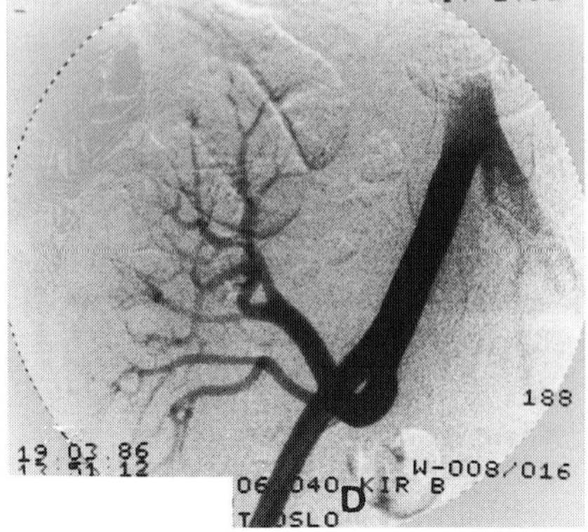

Fig. 7.5 A–D. Renal artery branch stenosis and aneurysms (**A**) treated with ex vivo excision of the affected portion of vessel (**B**) and revascularization (**C**) with grafts from the unaffected main renal artery (*ra*) and saphenous vein (*sv*). Radiographic appearance after autotransplantation to the right internal iliac artery (**D**). (From Brekke et al. 1992)

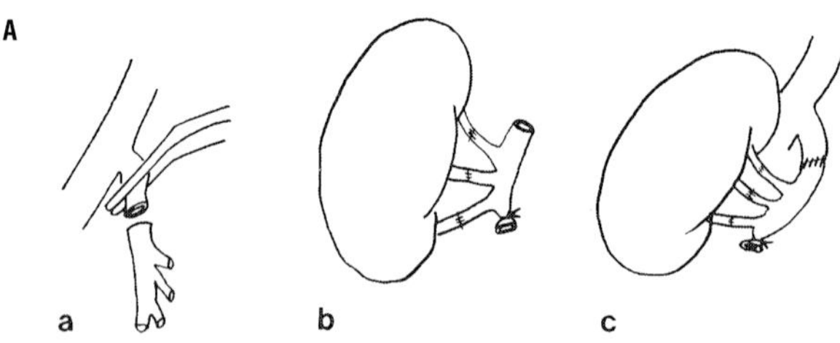

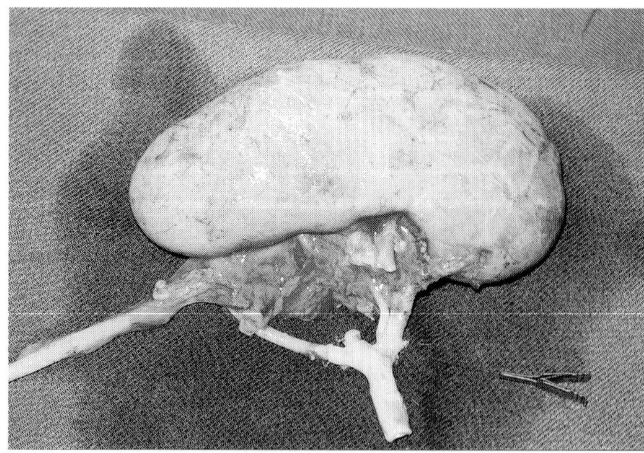

Fig. 7.6 A,B. Reconstruction of a main arterial trunk and three renal artery branches using autologous internal iliac artery alone (**A**) (from Brekke 1990) and in combination with the „double barrel" technique (**B**)

7.6
Renal Reimplantation and Postoperative Control

During bench surgery, a second team of surgeons has prepared the recipient site as described in Chap. 5. When the reconstruction is completed, the kidney is reimplanted to the ipsilateral iliac fossa, anastomosing the renal vein to the external iliac vein and the renal artery to the internal (Fig. 5.5) or external iliac artery (for technical details, see Chap. 5). Iliac endarterectomy may be required in patients with extensive atherosclerosis. Ureteroneocystostomy is accomplished by a modification of the method described by Paquin (Paquin 1959) (Fig. 5.6).

Total and split kidney function is assessed pre- and posttransplantation by creatinine measurements and isotope renograms. Unobstructed urinary flow is documented by urography and/or ultrasound examination. The potential deleterious effect of the contrast material on renal function implies that autotransplant arteriography should be performed to rule out autotransplant artery stenosis only in cases of postoperatively reduced autotransplant function or of de novo or persistent hypertension.

7.7
Results

The result of any treatment modality will depend, more or less, on patient selection. When comparing results of in situ and ex vivo renal artery repair, it can usually be presumed that ex vivo repair has been chosen for the most complex cases and that the results are, therefore, not directly comparable.

That ex vivo repair should be preferred for the treatment of renal artery aneurysms is demonstrated by the less favorable results published on in vivo surgery for this condition. In a recent series of 32 patients who underwent surgical treatment, 12 had either a total or partial nephrectomy, or a renal artery ligation. Renal artery reconstruction was performed in 20, of which seven were ex vivo. Blood pressure became normal in seven and remained unchanged in 15 (Dzsinich et al. 1993). This is in contrast to the functional survival of all 21 kidneys and the improvement of blood pressure in all patients in a series where all renal artery reconstructions where performed ex vivo (Brekke et al. 1992).

7.7.1
Effect on Hypertension

Large series of surgical renal revascularization have, in general, shown long-term clinical benefit in 70%–90% of patients, with a cure of hypertension in 30%–40% (Novick 1991; Poulias et al. 1991). Data from several centers on the effect on blood pressure of ex vivo vascular reconstruction are shown in Table 7.1, showing a cured-or-improved rate of 89%–100%. In our 56 pretransplant hypertensive patients followed-up for 1–10 years (mean 4.3), blood pressure was normalized or improved in 51 (91%). Thirty-seven were cured, i.e., became normotensive without antihypertensive drugs, while blood pressure was considerably reduced in 14. Hypertension was unaffected by the surgical intervention in five patients.

Table 7.1. Results of ex vivo repair of renal artery fibromuscular dysplasia. Effect on hypertension

Author	Number of kidneys	Cured	Improved	Cured or improved	Lost kidneys
Jordan 1985	14	13(93%)	1	14(100%)	
Dubernard 1985	33	27(81%)	5	32(97%)	
Kent 1987	45	34(75%)	6	40(89%)	
Novick 1991	54	45(83%)	9	54(100%)	
Barral 1992	15	11(73%)	4	15(100%)	2
Brekke 1992	56	37(66%)	14	51(91%)	2
Murray 1994	37	26(70%)	10	36(97%)	1

Table 7.2. Results of ex vivo repair of renal artery fibromuscular dysplasia. Effect on renal function

Author	Number of kidneys	Improved or unchanged	Lost kidneys
Lacombe 1989	41	85%	3
Novick 1991	61	89%	
Brekke 1992	63	95%	2
Murray 1994	48	100%	0

7.7.2
Effect on Kidney Function

Several authors have reported excellent results of ex vivo repair of renal artery FMD, with improvement or salvage of renal function in the majority of treated patients (Table 7.2). In our own series, 60 of 63 autotransplanted kidneys (95%) retained long-term function. One kidney was lost several months postoperatively due to progression of residual FMD, and vascular thrombosis occurred in two pediatric patients, both 2 years of age. No deterioration of autograft function was observed during long-term follow-up. Occurrence of FMD in the contralateral kidney was observed in four kidneys, of which two were successfully treated by sequential autotransplantation at 3- and 7-year intervals.

7.7.3
Surgical Complications

Complications related to nephrectomy, renal preservation, and transplantation will be of the same category as those seen after renal allotransplantation, i.e., artery obstruction, bleeding from anastomoses, and urinary leak (Amante and Kahan 1994). However, the rate of complications after allotransplantations is increased due to the obligatory immunosuppressive medication. On the other hand, nonuremic patients will not benefit from the platelet malfunction related to uremia, and thus the potential risk of transplant artery thrombosis will be increased, depending on the complexity of the reconstruction performed. For thrombosis prophylaxis, our routine is to give low molecular heparin or acetylsalicylic acid, 75 mg/day. As mentioned in Chap. 5, lymphoceles are extremely rare after renal autotransplantation.

7.7.4
Patient Survival

Surgical mortality is less than 1% in modern series of renal revascularization if aortic reconstruction is not performed, equivalent to the mortality rate for renal PTA (Novick 1991; Brekke et al. 1992; Soulen 1994).

7.8
Conclusion

Interdisciplinary cooperation between surgeons, nephrologists, and intervention radiologists is essential for all patients with renovascular hypertension or renal dysfunction caused by FMD. The disadvantages of medical antihypertensive treatment include its high cost and the possible side-effects of drugs to be taken over the lifetime of the patient, as well as the risks of progressive renal artery disease. Steps to eliminate the cause of hypertension should therefore be taken when no obvious contraindication is present.

During the last decade, PTA has gradually become the treatment of choice for stenotic lesions of the main renal artery. It is also increasingly being applied for branch stenoses, and the majority of renal FMD cases are now treated by PTA. However, complications requiring a surgical procedure occurred in 17% of patients in a recent study (Weibull et al. 1993) and, because of the need for late surgical intervention for recurrences after PTA, no significant difference in median cost was found between PTA and surgery in a comparative study over a 4-year period (Weibull et al. 1991). To avoid serious complications, it has been suggested that the routine use of PTA should be limited to stenoses of the main renal artery in patients with two functioning kidneys (Dean et al. 1987; Shifrin et al. 1991). Because simple, main artery FMDs are often treated in local hospitals, while the more complex cases are referred to specialized centers, the proportion of FMD cases unsuitable for PTA cannot be assessed from the reported series of patients. However, Novick (1991) considered as many as 30% of renal FMD cases unsuitable for PTA.

For patients with complex renal artery lesions unsuitable for PTA and for patients in whom renal artery PTA has been unsuccessful, surgical revascularization remains the treatment of choice. Whether the reconstruction should be performed in situ or extracorporeally must be decided by the complexity of the anomaly and the preference of the surgeon. However, bench surgery with autotransplantation is an extremely safe approach, which is given priority in centers where renal transplantations are routinely performed. The ability to perform extracorporeal microvascular repair of branch renal artery lesions has extended the feasibility of revascularization to patients who would have been considered inoperable or candidates for nephrectomy (Martinez et al. 1990). The advantages of performing extracorporeal repair of the kidney in such cases include optimal exposure and a bloodless field with the kidney protected from warm ischemia, allowing generous time for accurate repair work.

The results published by several centers demonstrate that ex vivo vascular reconstruction with renal autotransplantation is a safe and effective way to treat RVH and maximize the salvage of kidneys affected by complex arterial pathology inaccessible to PTA. For fibromuscular dysplasia occurring in young patients, whose life expectancy is usually long, this type of surgery provides excellent long-term functional and anatomical results. The procedure is associated with few serious complications and normalization or improvement of blood pressure as well as stabilization or improvement of renal function is achieved in 90%–100% of the patients.

References

Amante AJ, Kahan BD (1994) Technical complications of renal transplantation (review). Surg Clin North Am 74(5):1117–1131

Barral X, Gournier JP, Frering V, Favre JP, Berthoux F (1992) Dysplastic lesions of renal artery branches: late results of ex vivo repair. Ann Vasc Surg 6(3):225–231

Belzer FO, Raczkowski A (1982) Ex vivo renal artery reconstruction with autotransplantation. Surgery 92:642–645

Bloom PB, Viner ED, Mazala M, Jannetta PJ, Stieber AC, Simmons RL (1989) Treatment of loin pain hematuria syndrome by renal autotransplantation (review). Am J Med 87(2):228–232

Brekke IB (1990) Management of multiple renal transplant arteries. Transpl Int 3:241

Brekke IB, Sødal G, Jakobsen A, Bentdal O, Pfeffer P, Albrechtsen D, Flatmark A (1992) Fibro-muscular renal artery disease treated by extracorporeal vascular reconstruction and renal autotransplantation: short- and long-term results. Eur J Vasc Surg 6(5):471–476

Cerny JC, Chang CY, Fry WJ (1968) Renal artery aneurysms. Arch Surg 96(4):653–663

Cluzel P, Raynaud A, Beyssen B, Pagny JY, Gaux JC (1994) Stenoses of renal branch arteries in fibromuscular dysplasia: results of percutaneous transluminal angioplasty. Radiology 193(1):227–232

Cohen JR, Shamash FS (1987) Ruptured renal artery aneurysms during pregnancy. J Vasc Surg 6(1):51–59

Dean RH, Callis JT, Smith BM, Meacham PW (1987) Failed percutaneous transluminal renal angioplasty: experience with lesions requiring operative intervention. J Vasc Surg 6:301–307

Dillon MJ (1994) Renovascular hypertension (review). J Hum Hypertens 8(5):367–369

Dubernard JM, Martin X, Gelet A, Mongin D, Canton F, Tabib A (1985) Renal autotransplantation versus bypass techniques for renovascular hypertension. Surgery 97(5):529–534

Dzsinich C, Gloviczki P, McKusick MA, Pairolero PC, Bower TC, Hallett JJ, Cherry KJ (1993) Surgical management of renal artery aneurysm. Cardiovac Surg 1(3):243–247

Ekelund L, Gerlock J, Molin J, Smith C (1978) Roentgenologic appearance of fibromuscular dysplasia. Acta Radiol [Diagn] (Stockh) 19(3):433–446

Ertel B, Schmitt R, Helmberger T, Schnur KP (1994) The multilocular occlusive form of fibromuscular hyperplasia (in German). Radiologe 34(2):63–66

George B, Zerah M, Mourier KL, Gelbert F, Reizine D (1989) Ruptured intracranial aneurysms. The influence of sex and fibromuscular dysplasia upon prognosis. Acta Neurochir (Wien) 97(1–2):26–30

Hageman JH, Smith RF, Szilagyi E, Elliott JP (1978) Aneurysms of the renal artery: problems of prognosis and surgical management. Surgery 84(4):563–572

Halllwachs O, Vollmar J (1971) Complete occlusion of the renal artery: nephrectomy or revascularization? (in German). Dtsch Med Wochenschr 96:53–56

Harrison EJ, McCormack LJ (1971) Pathologic classification of renal arterial disease in renovascular hypertension. Mayo Clin Proc 46(3):161–167

Harrow BR, Sloane JA (1959) Aneurysm of renal artery: report of five cases. J Urol 81:35–41

Heffelfinger MJ, Holley KE, Harrison EG, Hunt JC (1970) Arterial fibromuscular dysplasia studied at autopsy. Am J Clin Pathol 54:274

Ippolito JJ, LeVeen HH (1960) Treatment of renal artery aneurysms. J Urol 83:10–15

Jordan ML, Novick AC, Cunningham RL (1985) The role of renal autotransplantation in pediatric and young adult patients with renal artery disease. J Vasc Surg 2(3):385–392

Kent KC, Salvatierra O, Reilly LM, Ehrenfeld WK, Goldstone J, Stoney RJ (1987) Evolving strategies for the repair of complex renovascular lesions. Ann Surg 202:272–278

Klinge J, Mali WP, Puijlaert CB, Geyskes GG, Becking WB, Feldberg MA (1989) Percutaneous transluminal renal angioplasty: initial and long-term results. Radiology 171(2):501–506

Lacombe M (1989) Ex situ surgical repair of complex lesions of the renal artery (in French). Chirurgie 115(9):631–635

Leadbetter WF, Burkland CE (1938) Hypertension in unilateral renal disease. J Urol 39:611–626

Lin WW, McGee GS, Patterson BK, Yao JS, Pearce WH (1992) Fibromuscular dysplasia of the brachial artery: a case report and review of the literature (review). J Vasc Surg 16(1):66–70

Little PJ, Sloper JS, de Wardener HE (1967) A syndrome of loin pain and hematuria associated with disease of peripheral renal arteries. Q J Med 36:253–259

Lüscher TF, Lie JT, Stanson AW, Houser OW, Hollier LH, Sheps SG (1987) Arterial fibromuscular dysplasia (review). Mayo Clin Proc 62(10):931–952

Martinez A, Novick AC, Cunningham R, Goormastic M (1990) Improved results of vascular reconstruction in pediatric and young adult patients with renovascular hypertension. J Urol 144:717–720

Maxwell MH, Bleifer KH, Franklin SS, Varady PD, Deegan C (1972) Cooperative study of renovascular hypertension. Demographic analysis of the study. JAMA 220:1195–1204

Murray SP, Kent C, Salvatierra O, Stoney RJ (1994) Complex branch renovascular disease: management options and late results. J Vasc Surg 20(3):338–345

Novick AC (1991) Management of renovascular disease. A surgical perspective (review). Circulation 83[Suppl I]:1167–1171

Paquin AJ (1959) Ureterovesical anastomosis. The description and evaluation of a technique. J Urol 82:573–583

Perona PG, Baker WH, Fresco R, Hano JE (1989) Successful revascularization of an occluded renal artery after prolonged anuria. J Vasc Surg 9(6):817–821

Poulias GE, Skoutas B, Doundoulakis N, Prombonas E, Haddad H, Papaioannou K, Sendekeya S (1991) Surgical treatment of renovascular hypertension and respective late results. A twenty years experience. J Cardiovasc Surg (Torino) 32(1):69–75

Poutasse EF (1975) Renal artery aneurysms. J Urol 113(4):443–449

Ritota P, Quirke TE, Keys RC, Byer A (1994) A rare association of fibromuscular dysplasia of the femoral artery with aneurysm and occlusion treated alternatively (review). J Cardiovasc Surg (Torino) 35(3):239–241

Scheil AGR, Ibels LS, Thomas MAB, Graham JC (1985) Renal autotransplantation for severe loinpain/hematuria syndrome. Lancet ii:1216–1217

Schievink WI, Bjornsson J, Piepgras DG (1994) Coexistence of fibromuscular dysplasia and cystic medial necrosis in a patient with Marfan's syndrome and bilateral carotid artery dissections. Stroke 25(12):2492–2496

Shifrin EG, Witz M, Morag B (1991) Revascularisation for a poorly functioning solitary kidney. Eur J Vasc Surg 5:421–423

Simon N, Franklin SS, Bleifer KH, Maxwell MH (1972) Clinical characteristics of renovascular hypertension. JAMA 220(9):1209 1218

Soulen MC (1994) Renal angioplasty: underutilized or overvalued? Radiology 193:19–21

Stanley JC (1984) Renal vascular disease and renovascular hypertension in children (review). Urol Clin North Am 11(3):451–463

Stanley JC (1994) The evolution of surgery for renovascular occlusive disease (review). Cardiovac Surg 2(2):195–202

Stanley JC, Gewertz BL, Bove EL, Sottiurai V, Fry WJ (1975) Arterial fibrodysplasia. Histopathologic character and current etiologic concepts. Arch Surg 110(5):561–566

Tegtmeyer CJ, Selby JB, Hartwell GD, Ayers C, Tegtmeyer V (1991) Results and complications of angioplasty in fibromuscular disease. Circulation 83[Suppl I]:155–161

Tham G, Ekelund L, Herrlin K, Lindstedt EL, Olin T, Bergentz SE (1983) Renal artery aneurysms. Natural history and prognosis. Ann Surg 197(3):348–352

Van Bockel JH, Van Schilfgaarde R, Van Brummelen P, Terpstra JL (1989) Long-term results of renal artery reconstruction with autogenous artery in patients with renovascular hyperetension. Eur J Vasc Surg 3:515–521

Weibull H, Bergqvist D, Bergentz SE, Jonsson K, Hulthen L, Manhem P (1993) Percutaneous transluminal renal angioplasty versus surgical reconstruction of atherosclerotic renal artery stenosis: a prospective randomized study. J Vasc Surg 18(5):841–850

Weibull H, Bergqvist D, Jendteg S, Lindgren B, Persson U, Jonsson K, Bergentz SE (1991) Clinical outcome and health care costs in renal revascularization–percutaneous transluminal renal angioplasty versus reconstructive surgery. Br J Surg 78(5):620– 624

Complicated Renal Calculous Disease Treated by Extracorporeal Surgery and Autotransplantation

Per F. Pfeffer, Helge Bondevik, and Gunnar Sødal

8.1
Introduction

While a variety of techniques for in situ surgical renal stone removal have been described and used for decades (Gil-Vernet 1965; Smith and Boyce 1968; Gibbons et al. 1976), extracorporeal stone removal with subsequent autotransplantation of the kidney has had few proponents (Gil-Vernet et al. 1975; Flatmark et al. 1977; Gelin 1977; Novick 1981). The technique was first reported by Gil-Vernet and collaborators in 1975 for treatment of relapsing renal calculi. In our extensive experience with renal autotransplantation on various indications (Flatmark et al. 1989; Bondevik et al. 1990; Brekke et al. 1992), urinary calculous disease was the indication in approximately one third of the patients (Flatmark et al. 1989).

During the last decade, new alternative surgical procedures have evolved, and a number of minimally invasive techniques have been developed for the removal of urinary tract calculi. Consequently, the majority of stones within the urinary tract can now be managed without open surgery, using extracorporeal shockwave lithotripsy (ESWL), percutaneous nephrolithotomy (PCNL), or ureteroscopy (URS). These techniques have recently been refined and may be used in combination, when indicated for more complex urinary calculi.

Since the first clinical experience with ESWL in the fragmentation of kidney stones, newer studies indicate that approximately 85% of simple renal calculi can be treated by this method alone (Chaussy et al. 1982; Fuchs and Chaussy 1987). Patients with staghorn calculi or other complex stone problems will probably require PCNL. Initial enthusiastic descriptions of PCNL, with reports of high success rates from large series of patients, led to the referral of increasingly complicated cases. This resulted in an increase in postoperative complications from 13.6% to 24% in a series of 1000 patients. At the same time, the number of patients rendered stone-free or left with small fragments after PCNL alone, decreased from 93% to 65% (Jones et al. 1990). A higher success rate has been achieved by combining PCNL and ESWL, yielding stone-free results of 85%-90% in skilled hands (Schulze et al. 1989).

However, residual stones are still a problem. Patients who are not rendered stone-free after these procedures remain infected and are likely to have recurrent stones, requiring open surgery.

8.2
Indications for Extracorporeal Surgery

The most common indications for extracorporeal renal calculi removal are severe symptoms or threatened renal function caused by staghorn calculi, chronic recurrent pyelocalyceal calculi, or complex calculi not otherwise accessible. The aim of the procedure is to remove all calculous material from the pyelocalyceal system and thus prevent recurrent stones, chronic infections, and deterioration of renal function. When the etiology of the calculi formation is such that further formation of calculous material must be anticipated, the aim of the treatment is to ensure free passage of the stones to the urinary bladder. However, subsequent to the introduction of alternative methods for removal of calculi during the 1980s, the number of cases requiring bench surgery decreased substantially.

In our own series of 97 patients treated between 1973 and 1985 for complicated calculous disease, with bench surgery on 108 kidneys (Table 8.1), the indications for extracorporeal surgery were large staghorn calculi in two thirds of the patients and multiple pyelocalyceal calculi in one third. A specific condition predisposing to stone formation could be detected in 32 of the patients (Table 8.2). Patient age ranged from 3 to 75 years (mean 46.1). One third of the patients were older than 60 years of age, three over 70. Four patients were children and three teenagers. Of the patients, 69% had a history of previous stone surgery and 52% of the autografted kidneys had been operated upon before, with the number of operations ranging from 1 to 11 (mean 1.8). Of the patients, 74% had chronic or recurrent urinary tract infections and 62% had an infection at the time of autotransplantation. Twenty-eight per cent of the patients had only one functioning kidney (Table 8.1). A nephrectomy had been performed previously in 19 of these patients, because of calculous disease in 14, tuberculosis in three, and carcinoma in two. In eight patients, the contralateral kidney function had been lost because of staghorn calculi and chronic infection. Renal nonfunction was verified by angiography and radionuclide scans demonstrating renal flow below 20 ml/min. Six of these eight kidneys were removed during or after the autotransplantation. In 60% of the patients undergoing renal autotransplantation, the contralateral kidney was functioning well.

Table 8.1. Preoperative characteristics of 97 patients treated with autotransplantation of 108 kidneys for urinary calculous disease

	Solitary kidney	Two kidneys	
	Autotx	Unilateral autotx	Bilateral autotx
No. of patients	27	59	11
Age, mean, in years (range)	52.6 (22-75)	42.5 (3-74)	50.1 (11-67)
Previous stone surgery	85%	63%	64%
Urinary tract infection	81%	69%	82%
Renal dysfunction[a]	74%	7%	55%
No. of kidneys	27	59	22
Staghorn calculus	70%	75%	68%
Multiple pyelocalyceal calculi	30%	25%	32%

[a] Serum creatinine above 130 μmol/l.

Bilateral autotransplantation was performed in 11% of the patients because of bilateral stone disease. This was done as a two-stage procedure. The time elapsing between the first and second procedure ranged from 1 to 26 months, with a mean of 11 months.

Since the mid 1980s, most patients with urinary calculous disease have been treated by minimally invasive procedures, and only the most complicated cases have been referred for bench surgery. Since 1986, we have performed 19 autotransplantations for renal calculi in 12 females and 7 males, with a mean age of 37 years. Fifteen patients had previously been treated with invasive stone surgery, and four had only one functioning kidney at the time of autotransplantation (Table 8.3). A total of five patients had a pre-operative diagnosis of medullary sponge kidneys, four patients had cystinuria, and one patient had oxalosis. The etiology of stone formation could not be determined in the remaining nine patients.

Table 8.2. Pathogenesis of stone formation in 32 patients treated with renal autotransplantation

Pathogenesis	No. of patients
Cystinuria	7
Primary hyperparathyroidism	6
Tuberculosis	4
Congenital medullary sponge kidney	3
Other congenital malformations	1
Ureteric stricture after previous surgery	3
Paraplegia	1
Idiopathic hypercalciuria	1
Prolonged steroid therapy	6
Total	32

Table 8.3. Pre- and postoperative data on 19 patients treated between 1986 and 1995 with autotransplantation for renal calculous disease

	Preoperatively (no. of pat.)	Postoperatively (no. of pat.)
Stone surgery	15	1
Solitary kidney	4	4
Urinary tract infection	12	1[*]
Renal dysfunction[a]	6	6
Staghorn calculus	7	0
Multiple pyelocalyceal calculi	14	6[**]

[*]after the initial postoperative period
[a] Serum creatinine above 130 µmol/l
[**]4 patients with medullary sponge kidneys , 1 cystinuria, 1 oxalosis

8.3
Preoperative Examination and Evaluation

Metabolic disorders and other conditions predisposing to calculi formation should be identified or excluded by appropriate measures.

When renal autotransplantation is planned, the following procedures will yield important information for the surgeon and for patient follow-up:

- Aortic angiography to visualize the number and position of renal arteries, artery stenoses when present, and possible pathology of the renal parenchyma. Gross aortoiliac pathology should be detected and preferably attended to before the auto-transplantation, as vascular surgery in this region at a later stage could put the auto-transplant in jeopardy.

– Urography to visualize the calyces, renal pelvis, and ureter.
– Radionuclide studies, with simultaneous estimation of the total effective renal plasma flow (ERPF) and the functional distribution between the right and left kidney. This also serves as a baseline for similar postoperative examinations. In patients with a single kidney, urea and creatinine will give sufficient information.
– Ultrasonography is performed when the angiogram has indicated renal parenchymal pathology. Renal parenchymal pathology may be further elucidated by computer tomography.
– Culturing of urine specimens to diagnose urinary tract infections. Patients with recent or current infections are treated aggressively pre-, per-, and postoperatively, according to standard guidelines. Patients with no history of urinary tract infection should receive antibiotic prophylaxis on the day of surgery.

8.4
Surgical Procedures

The kidney is routinely removed through a flank incision. Alternatively, a long midline incision permits both the removal and subsequent reimplantation of the kidney. According to our preference, the ureter is always transsected. The kidney is flushed and preserved in cold (4-10°C), low molecular weight dextran solution (Euro-Collins; Squifflet et al. 1981). Bench surgery is performed under hypothermia (Fig. 8.1). The procedure usually starts with a longitudinal incision in the renal pelvis, removing as much calculous material as possible through this approach (Fig. 8.2). The removal of large stones in the calyces may require incisions in calyceal necks, but this should be minimized to avoid parenchymal hemorrhage that may be difficult to control. Contraincisions in the parenchyma at the top of the usually dilated calyces facilitate stone removal. These nephrotomies are later closed with hemostatic, interrupted sutures. The importance of complete removal of all stones in the collecting system is stressed (Fig. 8.3). The removal of all calculous material is confirmed by fluoroscopic examinations (Fig. 8.4). Insertion of cannulae into the kidney parenchyma in two planes, under fluoroscopic guidance, will pinpoint stones that are hard to locate by palpating the kidney or hard to visualize through incisions already made in the parenchyma. This procedure is valuable in minimizing the number and extent of nephrotomies.

After bench surgery, the kidney is reimplanted extraperitoneally in the iliac region through a separate incision, using the standard procedure for renal allotransplantation as described in Chap. 5. If the autotransplant involves the patient's one remaining kidney, it is implanted on the contralateral side, so that the renal pelvis and ureter will lie in front of the renal vessels. If the contralateral kidney is preserved, the autotransplant is implanted on the ipsilateral side to prevent conflict with the ureter of the other kidney. Revascularization of the autotransplant is performed with conventional vascular techniques. The renal vein is anastomosed end-to-side to the external iliac vein. The renal artery is anastomosed either end-to-end to the internal iliac or end-to-side to the external iliac artery. Where bilateral autotransplantation is required, at least one of the kidneys should be anastomosed to the external iliac artery to avoid interruption of both internal iliac arteries, as this may lead to male impotence and gluteal pains due to circulatory insufficiency. A ureteroneocystostomy is constructed following renal revascularization. In patients with cystinuria or other disorders predisposing to

Fig. 8.1. Backtable surgery with the kidney submerged in ice water

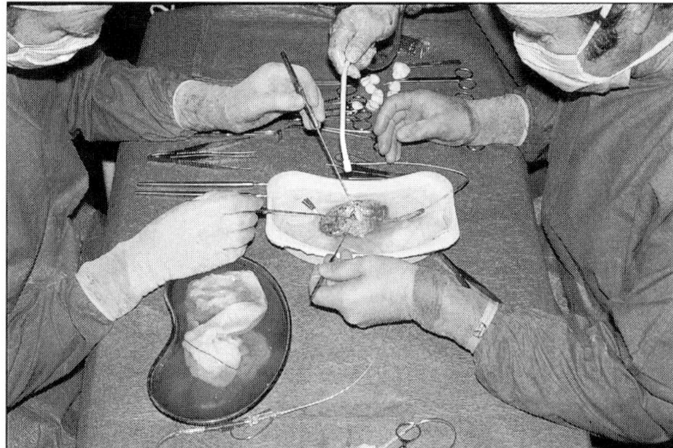

Fig. 8.2. Removal of calculi through an incision in the renal pelvis

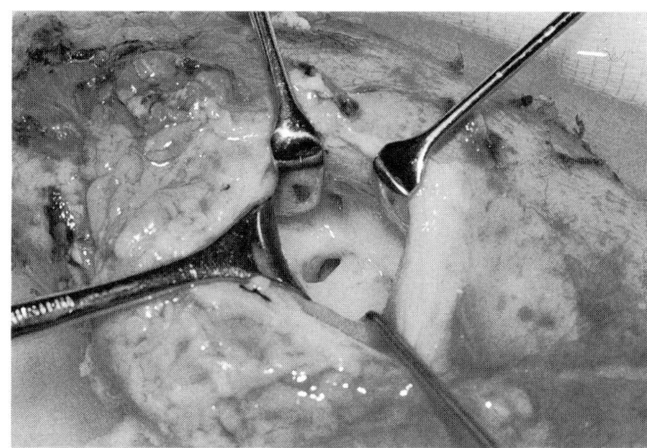

Fig. 8.3. Removal of all renal calculi often requires additional incisions in the renal parenchyma

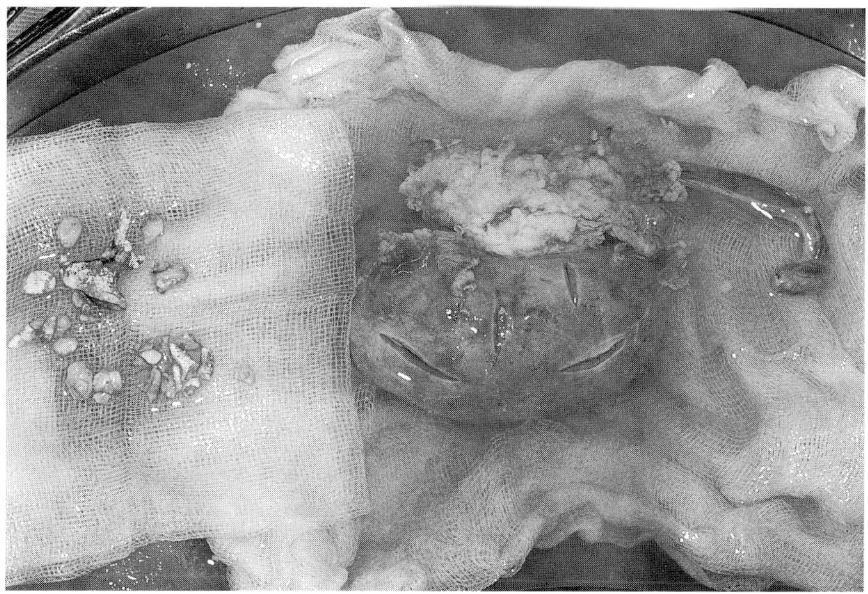

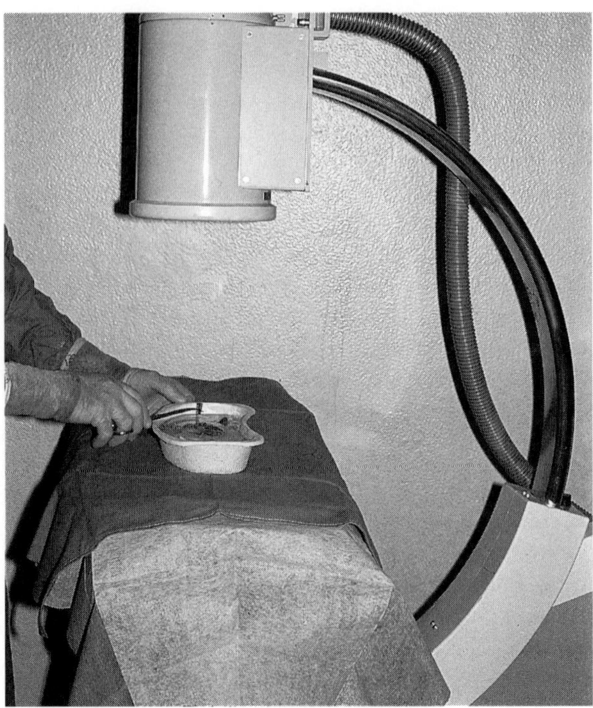

Fig. 8.4. Complete removal of calculi is ensured peroperatively by fluoroscopic examination, and hard to find residual stones are located with syringes in two planes

chronic recurrence of calculous formation, a pyelocystostomy should be constructed to ensure prompt discharge of newly formed calculous material (Pettersson et al. 1983). For this purpose, most of the extrarenal pelvis is excised, leaving enough tissue to ensure a wide anastomosis to the top of the bladder. This anastomosis is sewn in one layer with an interrupted 5-0 absorbable suture. Using this technique, emphasis is put on placing the kidney medially so that it can move with the bladder (Fig. 8.5). Otherwise, the kidney will fix the bladder laterally in a stretched position. This would increase the residual urine in the bladder and the risk of urinary infection. The renal artery, and the internal iliac artery to which it is anastomosed, should be relatively long to allow this placement of the kidney.

The pyelocystostomy also allows for extraction of calculous material directly from the renal pelvis with a cystoscope, if this should be necessary at a later stage.

Where stone extraction necessitates sharp dissection of the calyces or the renal parenchyma, a nephrostomy tube is routinely inserted, and continuous irrigation into the renal pelvis and out through the bladder catheter is started immediately before the graft is revascularized. This is required to prevent blood accumulation and clot formation in the calyces and renal pelvis.

When autotransplantation of both kidneys is indicated, this is done sequentially with the interval demanded by the clinical situation.

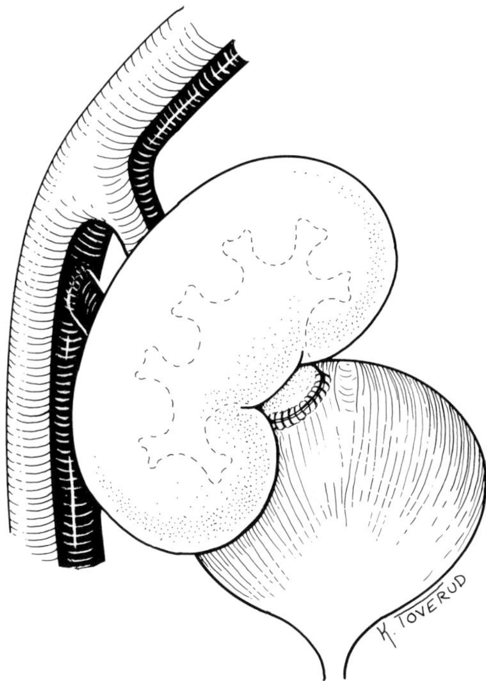

Fig. 8.5. A pyelocystostomy is constructed in chronic stone producers to allow free passage of stones to the urinary bladder.

8.5
Postoperative Follow-up

Irrigation through the nephrostomy tube is continued until the fluid from the bladder catheter is clear, usually 1-3 days postoperatively. When irrigation is stopped, the nephrostomy tube is connected to a closed drainage system. An antegrade pyelogram is performed to ensure free passage of urine to the bladder before the tube is removed. If residual thrombotic material is present in the collecting system, the pyelogram is repeated after some days. The urokinase present in the urine will usually dissolve the clot over a week or two. The tube is left in place until all clots have dissolved and to ensure that a channel has formed, which will prevent perinephric leakage of urine after tube removal. This requires a minimum of 2-3 weeks. Repeated urine cultures are taken during this time.

Renal radionuclide scans, intravenous pyelography, and duplex ultrasonography are routinely performed before discharge from hospital. The patients are readmitted at 3 and 12 months after the operation and at yearly intervals thereafter. Again, the function of the autotransplant (and of the in situ kidney when present) is investigated by radionuclide studies and intravenous pyelography. When a pyelocystostomy has been constructed, the pyelography will usually not give a very high concentration of contrast in the renal pelvis, because the urine will normally drain very rapidly into the bladder, thus confirming that the size of the anastomosis between the bladder and the

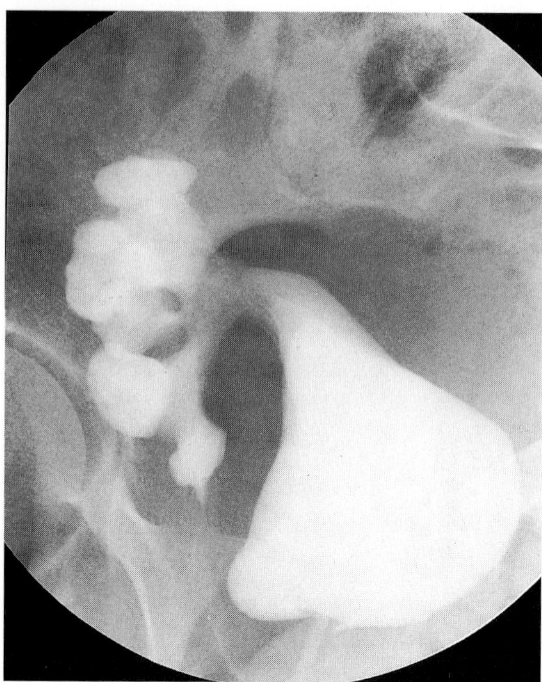

Fig. 8.6. Postoperative X-ray control of a pyelocystostomy through retrograde injection of contrast medium

renal pelvis is adequate. If required, a retrograde cystopyelography will give better visualization of the urinary tract (Fig. 8.6). Urine cultures are taken to identify possible urinary tract infections. After discharge, the patients should be followed up locally for urinary tract infections and renal function. The importance of high daily fluid intake is stressed.

The mean postoperative follow-up in our study was 3 years (range 1-12 years).

The cold ischemia time of the autotransplanted kidneys ranged from 1 to 6 h (mean 3.6). The surgical procedures lasted a total of 5-12 h (mean 8.3), and 0-21 units of blood (mean 4.3) were given. In patients with two kidneys, additional simultaneous nephrectomy of a nonfunctioning kidney was performed in five, while contralateral in situ pyelolithotomy was carried out in four patients. Additional surgery included pyeloplasty in three patients. Complete stone removal was not attempted in three patients with a total of four medullary sponge kidneys.

8.6
Results

Chronic or recurrent urinary tract infection had been a problem in 72 of our patients (74%) preoperatively. Of these patients, 50 (69%) were considered cured and another 12 (18%) improved during the follow-up period. Patients without preoperative infection remained free of infection during follow-up.

8.6.1
Recurrence of Calculi

Eighty-seven patients with 99 renal autografts were followed for more than 1 year after extracorporeal calculi removal. Recurrent calculi occured in one autograft only, while calculi were detected in the contralateral nonautografted kidney in six of 56 patients followed for more than 1 year after unilateral renal autotransplantation.

Two patients had tiny residual calculous fragments in the renal parenchyma after completion of extracorporeal surgery. These fragments neither increased in size nor gave symptoms during the observation period. Three patients developed a calculous cap on the ureteric nipple 3-9 months postoperatively. This was easily removed transurethrally with no subsequent recurrence. One of these patients, however, had impaired renal pelvic drainage and developed a frank recurrence of three small calculi in the renal pelvis 11 months after operation. Lithotomy and pyeloureteroplasty were performed, and the patient remained free of recurrence during further follow-up.

In three patients with four medullary sponge kidneys, complete clearance of stone material was not attempted, as the main aim of the operations was to secure easy passage to the bladder. A pyelocystostomy was constructed in 11 patients. Most of these patients continued to pass stones, but with virtually no discomfort.

Of the more complex cases treated after 1986, seven patients had recurring stone formation after surgery, of which four were diagnosed as having medullary sponge kidneys, one cystinuria, and one oxalosis, while one patient had stones in the renal parenchyma related to scar tissue after previous invasive surgery.

Five patients who were treated with autotransplantation because of debilitating pain related to their stone disease were all relieved of their chronic severe pain after surgery (Table 8.4). When some sporadic pain prevailed, it was related to discharge of stones through the urethra in chronic stone producers, while one patient had moderate pain in the nephrectomy incision.

Table 8.4. Renal autotransplantation for chronic, debilitating pain

Etiology of stone production	Number of patients with debilitating pain	
	Preoperatively	Postoperatively[a]
Medullary sponge kidneys	2	0
Cystinuria	1	0
Unknown	2	0
Total	5	0

[a] A pyelocystostomy was constructed in all patients

8.6.2
Autotransplant Function

Transient postoperative renal functional impairment was defined as a creatinine elevation of more than 50 μmol/l with a subsequent return to the preoperative level or lower. This could be assessed after 107 autotransplantations. Transient functional impairment was found after 29 operations (27%), mainly in patients with reduced preoperative function (43%), in contrast to 12% of those with normal preoperative renal function.

Long-term functional impairment was defined as a persistent serum creatinine elevation of more than 20% above the preoperative value. Of 87 patients who were alive and without kidney loss during follow-up, a lasting functional impairment was observed in 8%. Again, this was more often seen in patients with reduced preoperative renal function. Of patients who had a single kidney, 12 had normal and 24 elevated, preoperative creatinine (excluding two patients with early kidney loss). Eleven patients (92%) with normal preoperative values retained or improved their renal function. So did 19 of 24 patients (79%) with impaired preoperative function.

8.6.3
Postoperative Complications

Postoperative complications occurred in 33% of the operations. These include sudden unexpected death in one patient, respiratory distress requiring ventilatory support after the first postoperative day in eight (including two patients with myasthenia and five with bronchial asthma), pneumonia in 13, pancreatitis in one, peptic ulcer in two, venous leg thrombosis in two, wound infection in seven, and autograft artery stenosis or thrombosis in one and three, respectively. Leakage from the pyelocystostomy occured in three patients, pyeloureteric obstruction in two, fistula in three, and prolonged urinary tract hemorrhage in two patients.

Reoperation was required in 12% of the autotransplantations. These included graftectomy (2 cases), repair of arterial anastomosis (3), iliac vein thrombectomy (1), correction of pyeloureteric stricture (2), removal of a residual ureteric stump (1), peptic ulcer surgery (2), drainage of peripancreatic fluid accumulation (1), and tracheostomy (1).

8.6.3.1
Mortality

Three patients died of myocardial infarction within 45 days of the operation, two dying with functioning grafts and one after autograft loss. Two further patients died 5 and 14 months postoperatively, after loss of autotransplant function. Early and late mortality rates were thus 3.1% and 2.1%, respectively.

8.6.3.2
Kidney Loss

Five autotransplants (4.6%) lost function in the postoperative period. Another three grafts (2.8%) were lost during long-term follow-up. Of the eight kidneys lost, six were surgery-related losses (thrombosis, infection, and hemorrhage) and two were caused by recurrence of calculous disease.

8.7
Summary

The relatively few references to renal bench surgery and autotransplantion for the treatment of renal calculous disease in recent literature reflect the fact that the indication for this procedure has changed since the introduction of extracorporeal shockwave lithotripsy and percutaneous nephrolithotomy (Lindblad et al. 1993). Some authors suggest, however, that complete removal of large or difficult stones by these procedures is an unrealistic goal in many cases (Lam et al. 1992; Holmes and Whitfield 1993). Several reports indicate that incomplete removal of renal calculi frequently leads to persistence of bacteriuria and early stone recurrence (Patterson et al. 1987; Segura 1990). The same authors conclude that 90% of the patients who were stone-free at discharge remained so. Extracorporeal backtable surgery on kidneys with large staghorn calculi or multiple stones allows for meticulous removal of calculous material with immediate X-ray documentation and for further exploration, if necessary. In our series of 108 autotranplantations performed for urinary calculous disease between 1973 and 1985, only 1% of the patients followed for more than 1 year postoperatively had recurrence of calculous material in the autotransplant. Patients who were free of urinary tract infection prior to surgery remained so in the follow-up period and, of those with infection at the time of surgery, 69% were cured and 18% improved after the procedure.

In the period after 1985, when only the most complicated cases were referred for autotransplantation, 12 of 19 patients had a history of chronic urinary tract infection prior to surgery. Four of these had bacteriuria after the initial postoperative period. Of those with postoperative infections, two were chronic stone producers, while one had a stone in the parenchyma related to scar tissue after previous treatment attempts.

Since 1986, the main indication for autotransplantation in 26% of our patients was recurrent chronic stone formation with disabling pain. None of these patients had severe pain in the autotransplanted kidney after surgery.

We conclude that renal autotransplantation is still a very valuable procedure in selected groups of patients with urinary calculous disease inaccessible to other treatment modalities.

References

Bondevik H, Albrechtsen D, Sødal G, Jakobsen A, Brekke I, Flatmark A (1990) Extracorporeal surgery and autotransplantation for complicated renal calculous disease in 108 kidneys. Scand J Urol Nephrol 24:307-313

Brekke IB, Sødal G, Jakobsen A, Bentdal O, Pfeffer P, Albrechtsen D, Flatmark A (1992) Fibro-muscular renal artery disease treated by extracorporeal vascular reconstruction and renal autotransplantation: short- and long-term results. Eur J Vasc Surg 6(5):471-476

Chaussy C, Schmidt E, Jocham D, Brendal W, Forssmann B, Walter V (1982) First clinical experience with extracorporally induced destruction of kidney stones by shock waves. J Urol 127:417-420

Flatmark A, Sødal G, Jervell J, Brodwall E, Enge I (1977) Preliminary experience with extracorporeal renal surgery and autotransplantation. Eur Surg Res 9:235-251

Flatmark A, Albrechtsen D, Sødal G, Bondevik H, Jakobsen JRA, Brekke I (1989) Renal autotransplantation. World J Surg 13(2):206-210

Fuchs G, Chaussy C (1987) ESWL for staghorn disease. Reassessment of our treatment strategy. World J Urol 5:237-244

Gelin LE (1977) Extracorporeal surgery for renal problems. Surg Ann 9(351):351-79

Gibbons R, Correa R Jr, Cummings K, Mason J (1976) Surgical management of renal lesions using in situ hypothermia and ischemia. J Urol 115:12-17

Gil-Vernet J (1965) New surgical concept of removing renal calculi. Urol Int 20:255-288

Gil-Vernet JM, Caralps A, Revert L, Andreu J, Carretero P, Figuls J (1975) Extracorporeal renal surgery. Workbench surgery. Urology 5:444-451

Holmes SA, Whitfield HN (1993) Management of complex renal calculi (review). World J Urol 11(1):31-36

Jones D, Russel G, Kellet M, Wickham J (1990) The changing practice of percutaneous stone surgery. Review of 1000 cases 1981-1988. Brit J Urol 66:1-5

Lam HS, Lingeman JE, Mosbaugh PG, Steele RE, Knapp PM, Scott JW, Newman DM (1992) Evolution of the technique of combination therapy for staghorn calculi: a decreasing role for extracorporeal shock wave lithotripsy. J Urol 148:1058-1062

Lindblad B, Bergqvist D, Kristiansen P (1993) Bilateral renal autotransplantation with direct pyelo-cystostomy in a patient with frequent disabling nephroureterolithiasis. Case report. Scand J Urol Nephrol 27(3):413-414

Novick AC (1981) Role of bench surgery and autotransplantation in renal calculous disease. Urol Clin North Am 8(2):299-312

Patterson DE, Segura JW, LeRoy AJ (1987) Long-term follow-up of patients treated by percutaneous ultrasonic lithotripsy for struvite staghorn calculi. J Endourol 1:177-180

Pettersson S, Brynger H, Henriksson C, Nilson AE, Ranch T (1983) Autologous renal transplantation with direct pyelocystostomy in the treatment of recurrent renal calculi. Br J Urol 55(2):154-161

Schulze H, Hertle L, Kutta A, Graff J, Senge T (1989) Critical evaluation of treatment of staghorn calculi by percutaneous nephrolithotomy and extracorporeal shock wave lithotripsy. J Urol 141:822-825

Segura JW (1990) Current surgical approaches to nephrolithiasis. Endocrinol Metab Clin of North Am 19:919-935

Smith M, Boyce W (1968) Anatropic nephrolithotomy and plastic calyrrhaphy. J Urol 99:521-527

Squifflet J, Pirson Y, Gianello P, Van Cangh P, Alexandre G (1981) Safe preservation of human renal cadaver transplants by Euro-Collins solution up to 50 hours. Transplant Proc 13:693-696

Ex Vivo Renal Resection and Autotransplantation for Renal and Urothelial Carcinoma

Gunnar Sødal, Øystein Bentdal, and Audun Flatmark

9.1
Introduction

In 1966 Scott reported on an attempt to remove a renal tumor at a sidetable, but the renal remnant proved to be insufficient for reimplantation (Scott 1966). From the early 1970s there are case reports about successful bench surgery treatment of renal (Calne 1971; Gelin et al. 1971; Flatmark et al. 1977) and urothelial carcinomas (Rhame 1973; Pettersson et al. 1979). Bench surgery and subsequent renal autotransplantation was shown to be a valid alternative to radical nephrectomy in selected patients with bilateral renal neoplasms or when malignancy occurs in a solitary kidney. However, only a few centers have reported more than ten cases (Rohl et al. 1979; Jacobs et al. 1980; Flatmark et al. 1989; Novick et al. 1990; Stormont et al. 1992), and large series are still lacking.

9.2
Indications for Extracorporeal Surgery

Radical nephrectomy is the standard surgical procedure for the treatment of renal carcinoma (de Kernion 1986). This procedure implies the excision of Gerotas fascia and its contents, including the kidney and the adrenal gland. Nephroureterectomy including resection of a bladder cuff is the recommended procedure for pelvic or ureteral tumors (Droller 1986). In patients with a solitary kidney or bilateral neoplasms, these procedures will obviously make the patient uremic. They will be dependent on dialysis, and renal allotransplantation may subsequently be required. Therefore, several authors have advocated a more conservative surgical approach, either by in situ tumor excision, with or without cooling (Wickham 1975; Gibbons et al. 1976; Smith et al. 1984), or by extracorporeal resection and renal autotransplantation (Calne 1973; Flatmark et al. 1977; Pettersson et al. 1981). Most of the smaller renal carcinomas, especially those located at the poles, can be treated by in situ excision, but the larger tumors involving the central part of the kidney should be considered for extracorporeal renal resection and autotransplantation.

9.3
Surgical Technique

General aspects concerning surgical techniques are discussed in Chap. 5 and a detailed description of the nephrectomy procedure is given in Chap. 4.

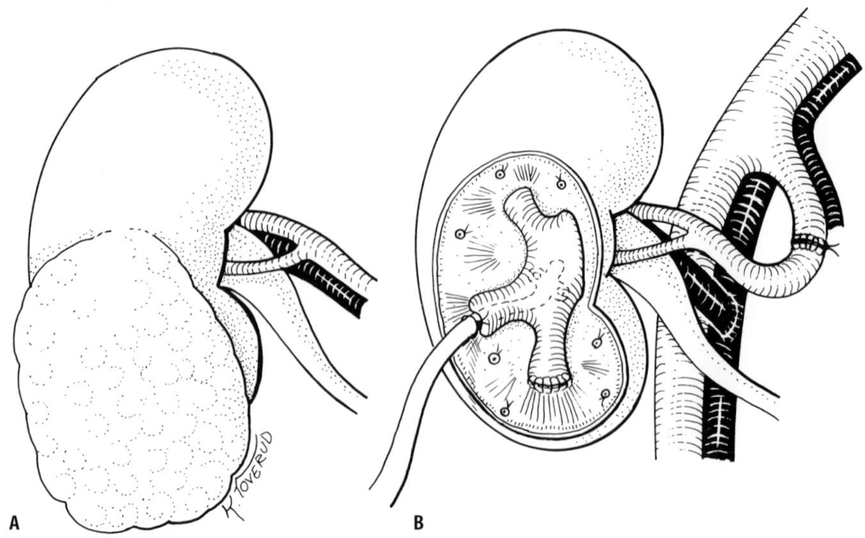

Fig. 9.1A,B. Drawing of a kidney showing a tumor involving the lower posterior portion (A). After ex vivo excision of the tumor, the kidney is transplanted to the right iliac fossa. A catheter is placed in one of the two transected calyces. The other one is closed by sutures (B)

9.3.1
Preparation of the Kidney (Bench Surgery)

The preparation of the kidney after nephrectomy is performed with the kidney in a basin with slushed ice. Gerota's fascia and the pernephric fat are removed and examined for carcinoma infiltration or metastasis.

9.3.1.1
Renal Carcinoma

The tumor, which in our experience is always visible on the surface of the kidney, is circumcised through the renal capsule 5-10 mm from the tumor. Further dissection is performed close to the well-defined pseudocapsule surrounding the tumor. After removal of the tumor, serial biopsies are provided from the resection area for histological examination of frozen sections to ensure tumor-free margins.

One or more calyces are commonly severed during this procedure. If so, a Mallecot catheter is introduced through one calyx into the renal pelvis in order to ensure safe drainage of urine (Fig. 9.1). Additional severed calyces have to be closed by sutures. The resection area is examined with magnifying glasses and all visible cut vessels are sutured in order to ensure good hemostasis. As illustrated in Figs. 9.1 and 9.2D, the tumor bed is commonly left open, accessible for extra hemostatic stitches if bleeding occurs after revascularization of the kidney. In some cases the tumor bed may be closed with parenchymal sutures as shown in Fig. 9.3.

The replantation of the kidney is done according to the description in Chap. 5.

Fig. 9.2 A-D. Asynchronously occurring bilateral renal carcinoma in a 50-year-old man. Computer tomography (January 1994) showing a large tumor in the left kidney. This was treated by nephrectomy (A). Computer tomography (May 1995) showing central tumor in the right kidney (B, C). Ex vivo extirpation of the tumor. The tumor bed is left open (D)

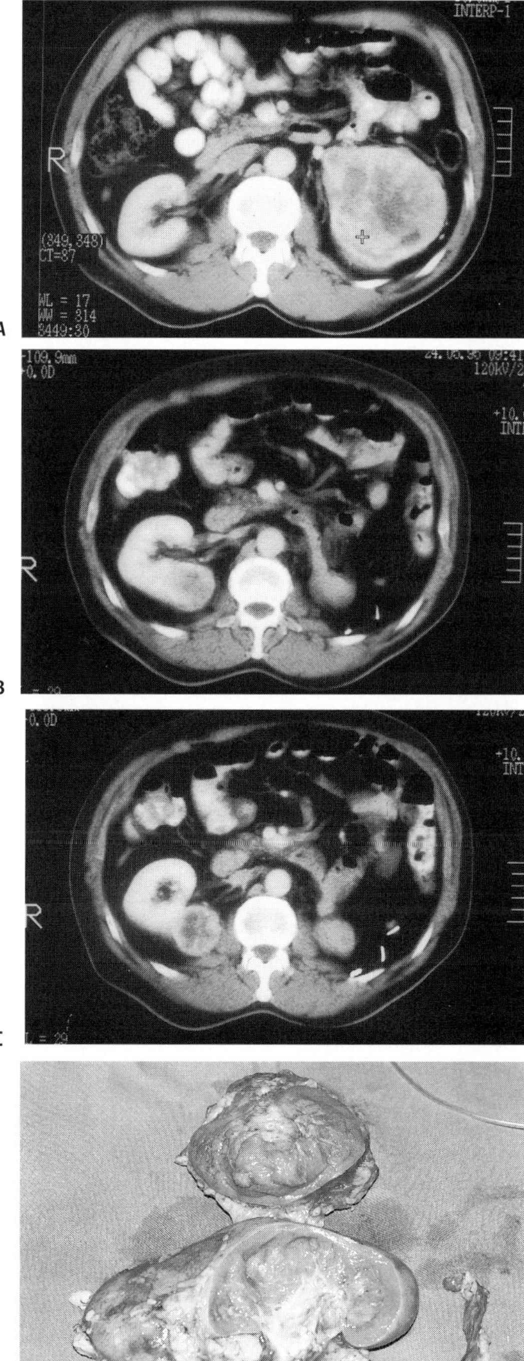

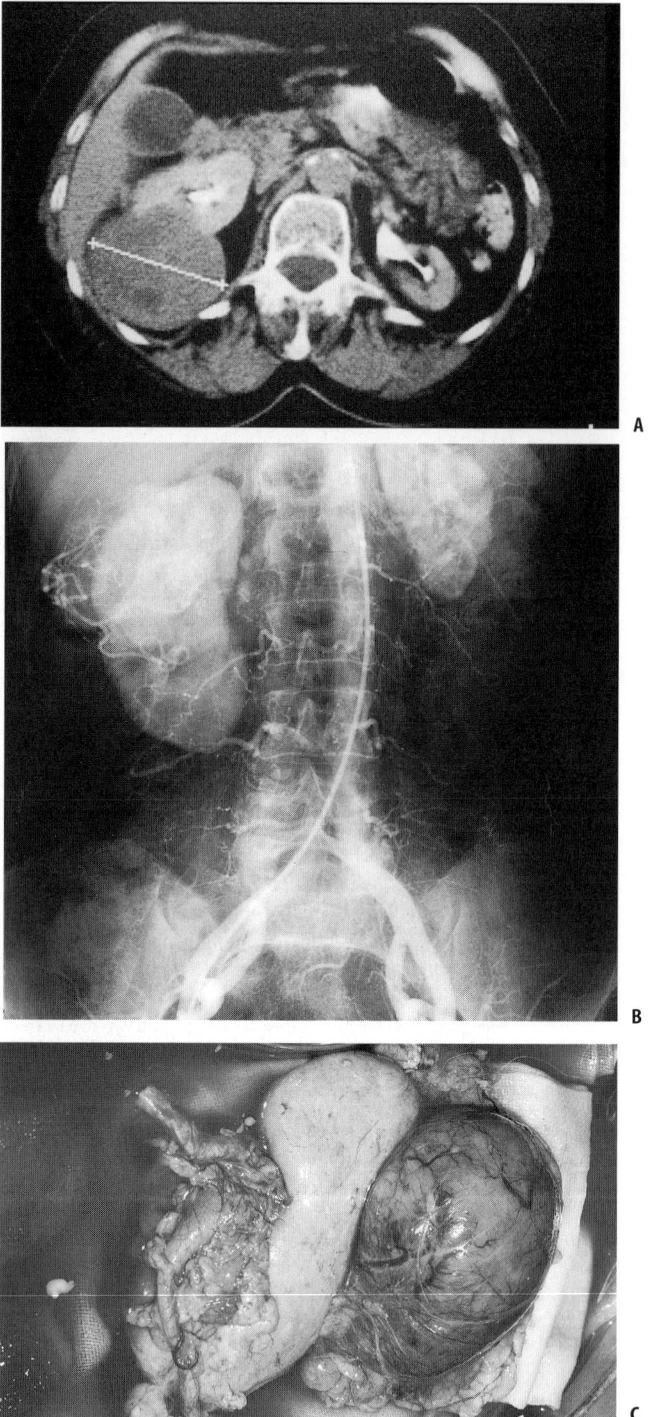

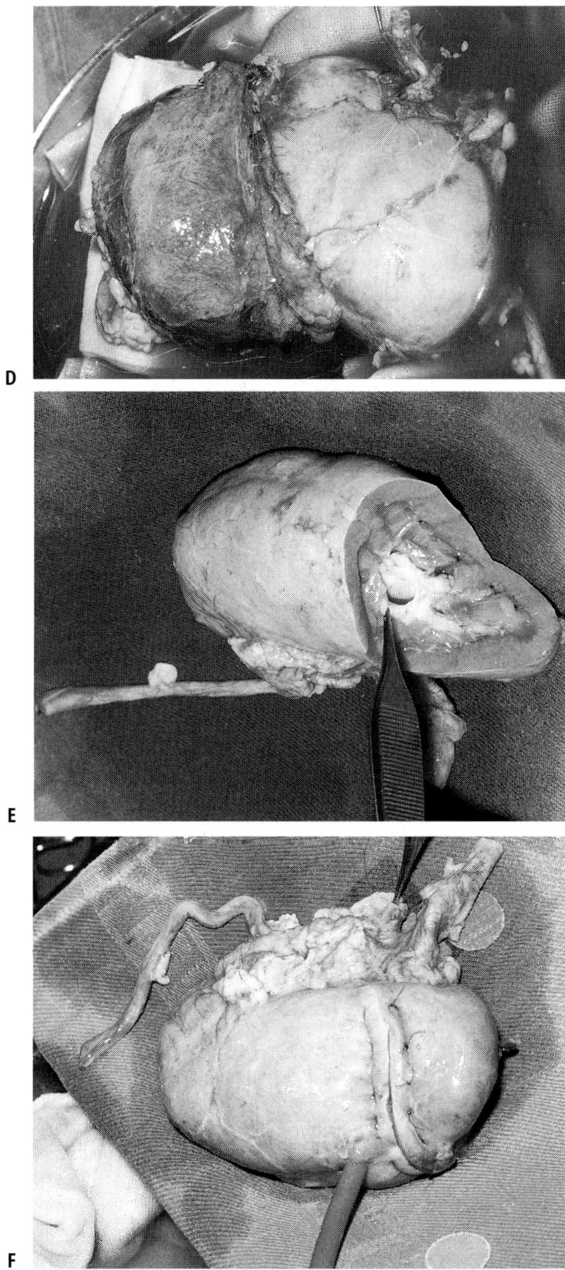

Fig. 9.3 A-F. Computer tomography (A) and angiography (B) in a 73-year-old woman, showing a hypoplastic left kidney and a large carcinoma involving the posterior portion of a normally sized right kidney. Ex vivo posterior (C) and anterior (D) view of the right kidney before removal of the tumor. Posterior view of the kidney after removal of the tumor (E). The resection bed is closed by sutures, and a nephrostomy catheter is placed in the pelvis for drainage of urine (F)

9.3.1.2
Urothelial Carcinoma

In patients with urothelial carcinoma of the renal pelvis or ureter, the kidney and ureter with a cuff of the bladder is removed en bloc as described in detail in Chap. 4. The nephroureterectomy is followed by extracorporeal removal of the ureter and as much as possible of the renal pelvis, at a safe distance from the tumor. The brim of the renal pelvis is anastomosed to the top of the bladder after revascularization of the kidney, as described in Chap. 8. This technique facilitates the examination of the renal pelvis and calyces by a flexible cystoscope after the operation. A postoperative cystopyelogram should demonstrate a wide passage between the bladder and renal pelvis (Fig. 9.4B).

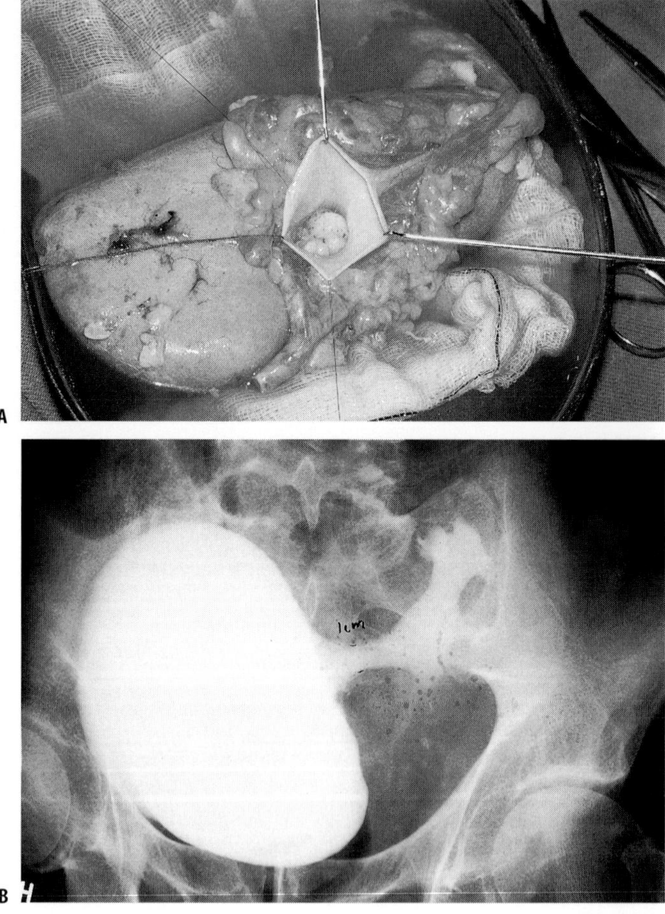

Fig. 9.4 A,B. Ex vivo extirpation of urothelial carcinoma located in the right renal pelvis of a 55-year-old man. Left nephroureterctomy had been performed in 1972 for urothelial carcinoma in the left ureter. With the right kidney on the backtable, the tumor is visualized in the renal pelvis before tumor excision is performed (A). A cystopyelogram postoperatively demonstrates a wide opening between the bladder and pelvis (B)

9.4
Postoperative Follow-up

Patients treated for renal carcinoma should be readmitted every 6 months and examined for metastases or recurrent tumor in the autografted kidney. Computer tomography of the kidney, liver, and the retroperitoneal space, as well as an X-ray examination of the lungs, are performed. An autograft angiography is performed if the computer tomography is inconclusive regarding recurrence of tumor in the transplanted kidney.

Urethracysto-pyeloscopy is routine in patients treated for urothelial carcinoma. Recurrent tumors in the bladder, pelvis, or calyces are treated by transurethral resection. These patients should be seen more frequently for reexamination and treatment.

A thorough physical examination, routine blood analysis, and cytological and bacteriological examination of the urine should be done at every follow-up.

9.5
Own Experience

Patients with carcinomas found unsuitable for in situ excision by the urologists have been referred to our transplant unit for ex vivo surgery and renal autotransplantation since 1975. By the end of 1995, 42 autotransplantations had been performed, 31 for renal carcinomas and 11 for urothelial carcinomas.

There were 23 males and eight females with renal carcinoma. Their ages ranged from 49 to 75 years (median 66 years). Eleven patients had bilateral carcinomas, while 20 patients developed carcinomas in a solitary kidney. Ten patients had lost a kidney due to carcinoma 1 to 16 (median 4) years earlier, and ten kidneys were lost for other reasons (Table 9.1).

Table 9.1. Basis for contralateral kidney nonfunction or nephrectomy in 42 patients referred for extracorporeal surgery for renal and urothelial carcinoma

Basis for contralateral nephrectomy/nonfunction	Renal carcinoma group (n=31)	Urothelial carcinoma group (n=11)
Asynchronous carcinoma	10	3
Infection	5	3
Agenesia	1	2
„Nonfunctioning" kidney	4	
Synchronous carcinoma*	11	3

* Bilateral renal involvement at the time of surgery

Two females and nine males were treated for urothelial carcinoma, ten in the renal pelvis and one in the ureter. Patient age ranged from 47 to 73 years (median 55 years). Three patients had urothelial carcinoma in both kidneys and eight developed carcinoma in a solitary kidney. The reason for kidney loss in the patients with a solitary kidney was urothelial carcinoma in two, renal carcinoma in one, and other causes in five (Table 9.1). Three of the patients had previously been treated by transurethral resection for recurring bladder papillomas.

In all 14 patients with bilateral carcinomas, the best kidney was autografted, while the contralateral kidney was removed .

One patient had been operated for carcinoma of colon 2 years prior to autotransplantation. Six patients with renal carcinoma and one with urothelial tumor were on medical treatment for hypertension. Ten of the patients with renal carcinoma and five of the patients with urothelial carcinoma had impaired renal function with serum creatinine higher than 125 µmol/l (Tables 9.2 and 9.3).

Table 9.2. Renal function in 31 patients treated for renal carcinoma

	Serum creatinine µmol/l		Patients with serum creatinine >125 µmol/l (n)
	Range	Median	
Preoperative	75-156	119	10
Postoperative	80-330	160	20

Table 9.3. Renal function in 11 patients treated for urothelial carcinoma

	Serum creatinine µmol/l		No. of patients with serum creatinine > 125 µmol/l (n)
	Range	Median	
Preoperative	79-200	122	5
Postoperative	76-175	124	5

The ureter could be spared for neoureterocystostomy in most cases of renal carcinoma, but in three patients the ureter and part of the renal pelvis had to be removed together with the tumor situated in the lower pole of the kidney. The brim of the renal pelvis and calyx was anastomosed directly to the top of the bladder according to the technique described for urothelial carcinoma.

9.6
Results

9.6.1
Perioperative Complications

Two patients treated for renal carcinoma died 6 and 8 weeks postoperatively, both of septicemia, initiated by urinary leakage and pneumonia, respectively. The latter patient also had secondary amyloidosis due to chronic rheumatoid arthritis.

Surgical reintervention was required in three patients treated for renal carcinomas. One patient had a renal vein thrombosis with anuria a few hours after the autotransplantation. After thrombectomy and temporary hemodialysis for 2 weeks, he regained a reduced renal function with serum creatinine of 330 µmol/l. Percutaneous pyelostomy drainage had to be established for 1 week in one patient with a pelvic hemorrhage and obstruction of the ureter by blood clots. The third patient had a stricture of the ureter caused by periureteral fibrosis 3 months after autotransplantation. Reoperation with ureterolysis was successful.

9.6.2
Long-Term Results

9.6.2.1
Renal Carcinoma

Recurrence of tumor in the graft was observed in five patients 6 to 40 months (median 11 months) after autotransplantation (Table 9.4), and four of the grafts were subsequently removed. Two of these patients received a kidney allotransplant after 1 year on hemodialysis. One of them had excellent graft function, but died 4 years later of metastases, 8 years after the autotransplantation. The other patient had an early irreversible rejection and died of septicemia 5 years after the autotransplantation. One patient developed metastases after graftectomy and died 1 year later, while the fourth one is still on hemodialysis waiting for a renal allotransplant. The fifth patient developed lung metastases as well as recurrence of tumor in the graft. He is still alive with adequate renal function 28 months after autotransplantation.

Table 9.4. Clinical data on 42 patients with renal or urothelial carcinoma who underwent extracorporeal tumor excision and renal autotransplantation

Tumor histology	Number	Mean patient age (years)	Recurrence of tumor in the graft	Occurrence of metastasis	Death caused by tumor	Presently alive
Renal carcinoma	31	66	5	14	11	15
Urothelial carcinoma	11	55	4	3	3	7

Metastases occurred in 14 of the 29 surviving patients operated for renal carcinoma (Table 9.4). Retrospectively, two of these patients had detectable metastasis at the time of operation. Eleven of them died 7 to 90 months (median 24) after the autotransplantation, giving a cancer mortality of 48.2%. Two patients are alive with metastases 20 and 28 months posttransplant. Lung resection with removal of two metastases was performed in one patient 9 months after autotransplantation. This patient is still without cancer recurrence 24 months later.

Five other patients died of other causes. In addition to the two patients who died postoperatively, two more patients died without tumor recurrence 6 and 8 years after autotransplantation. The fifth patient died of septicemia after renal allotransplantation. Thirteen patients are alive and free from carcinoma, 12 to 127 months (median 68 months) after autotransplantation.

Renal function was moderately impaired after autotransplantation (Table 9.2). Two thirds of the patients had a postoperative serum creatinine above 125 μmol/l compared to one third preoperatively. The median serum creatinine increased from 119 to

160 µmol/l. Five of the six patients, who had hypertension prior to operation, were normotensive postoperatively. Only one required antihypertensive drugs.

9.6.2.2
Urothelial Carcinoma

Recurrence of tumors in the renal pelvis and bladder occurred in four of the patients within 1 year posttransplant. Carcinoma infiltration of the kidney and perirenal tissue occurred in one of them 24 months posttransplant. A nephrocystoprostatectomy was performed, but the patient died 6 months later because of liver metastases. No invasive growth was observed in the other three patients, and the recurrent tumors have been treated by transurethral resection. Contralateral nephroureterectomy had been carried out 10 years prior to autotransplantation in one of them. However, the intramural part of the ureter had not been removed, and the 2 cm long ureter stump was the origin of a tumor requiring surgical bladder resection. Four patients had no recurrence of tumor.

Three of the 11 patients operated for urothelial carcinoma developed metastasis and died 9, 12 and 30 months after the operation, respectively, giving a cancer mortality of 27.2%. A fourth patient died because of prostatic carcinoma with metastases 32 months posttransplant

Renal function was unchanged postoperatively (Table 9.3) and only the one patient who had already required antihypertensive drugs before the operation needed antihypertensive treatment postoperatively. Recurrence of tumor or metastasis related to the nephroureterectomy wound has not been observed.

9.7
Summary

Previous publications on extracorporeal renal neoplasm surgery have demonstrated primary graft loss due to acute irreversible tubular necrosis in 14% (Novick et al. 1990) and vascular thrombosis in 25% of cases (Stormont et al. 1992). In our series, renal function was preserved in all 42 patients. Only one patient needed temporary hemodialysis for 2 weeks. Two high-risk patients died 6 and 8 weeks postoperatively of septicemia, giving an early mortality rate of 4.7%. There were few other postoperative complications. This demonstrates that extracorporeal excision of renal and urothelial carcinoma combined with autotransplantation is a safe surgical procedure.

Sixteen percent of our patients treated for renal carcinoma had a recurrent tumor in the graft. Others have reported recurrence rates of 25% (Stormont et al. 1992). Recurrent tumors in the kidney remnant have been reported to occur in 3%-13% after in situ ennucleation or excision of renal carcinomas (Topley et al. 1984; Zincke et al. 1985; Morgan and Zincke 1990). This difference in recurrence rates is most likely explained by differences in patient selection. Small tumors, especially those located at the poles, are treated by in situ ennucleation or resection, while the larger tumors, involving the central part of the kidney, are referred for extracorporeal surgery.

Distant metastasis after treatment for renal cancer occurred in 14 patients, and 11 of them died 7-90 months (median 24 months) after autotransplantation. An additional three patients died 5, 6, and 8 years after autotransplantation, of septicemia, intestinal strangulation, and cardiac infarction, respectively. The fact that no local tumor recurrence at the nephrectomy site was observed indicates that all relapses were caused by undetectable subclinical metastasis present at the time of operation. The kidney-preserving autotransplantation procedure was thus very beneficial for these patients in terms of preservation of normal renal function throughout life. Radical nephrectomy would not have cured their malignancy, but dialysis treatment would have been required for the rest of their lives.

Most renal carcinoma patients are elderly and less than ideal candidates for renal allotransplantion, and kidney allografts are short in supply. This underlines the importance of considering alternatives to conventional nephrectomy in patients with a solitary kidney. Ex vivo repair and renal autotransplantation is a safe procedure, both regarding conservation of renal function and radical excision of the tumor. The importance of careful follow-up to detect tumor relapse in the kidney is emphasized. Tumor relapse has to be treated by graftectomy and hemodialysis, and allotransplantation must be considered if metastasis does not occur during a follow-up period of 1 year.

The autotransplantation technique provides a unique opportunity for combining a radical nephroureterectomy with a maximal excision of urothelial tissue in patients with urothelial cancer. Construction of a pyelocystostomy also facilitates the examination of the renal pelvis and calyces and the excision of recurrent tumors by urethracystopyeloscopy. It is mandatory to use a flexible scope for inspection of all calyces.

The patient with urothelial cancer is usually somewhat younger and better suited for allotransplantation. Therefore, if a urothelioma, relapsing in the follow-up period after autotransplantation, shows increasingly malignant degeneration, we advocate an aggressive treatment policy of early nephrocystectomy before metastases develop. After a period of hemodialysis the definite treatment will be allotransplantation with urinary drainage to a Bricker bladder.

Even though new technology expands the possibility of treating tumors in the ureter and the renal pelvis primarily by direct ureteroscopy, ex vivo surgical repair with autotransplantation is a sound and logical procedure for the treatment of renal tumors and urothelial cancer in patients with a solitary kidney or with bilateral involvement.

References

Calne RY (1971) Tumour in a single kidney: nephrectomy, excision, and autotransplantation. Lancet 2:761-762

Calne RY (1973) Treatment of bilateral hypernephromas by nephrectomy, excision of tumor, and autotransplantation. Lancet 2:1164-1167

de Kernion JB (1986) Renal tumors. In: Walsh PC, Gittes RE, Perlmutter AD, Stamey TA (eds). Campbell's Urology. Saunders, Philadelphia

Droller MJ (1986) Transitional cell cancer. Upper tracts and bladder. In: Walsh PC, Gittes RE, Perlmutter AD, Stamey TA (eds). Campbell's Urology. Saunders, Philadelphia

Flatmark A, Sødal G, Jervell J, Broadwall E, Enge I (1977) Preliminary experience with extracorporeal renal surgery and autotransplantation. Eur Surg Res 9:235-251

Flatmark A, Albrechtsen D, Sødal G, Bondevik H, Jakobsen A, Brekke IB (1989) Renal autotransplantation. World J Surg 13:206-210

Gelin LE, Claes G, Gustafsson </A>, Storm B (1971) Total bloodlessness for extracorporeal organ repair. Rev Surg 28:305-316

Gibbons RP, Correa RJ, Cummings KB, Mason JT (1976) Surgical management of renal lesions using in situ hypothermia and ischemia. J Urol 115:12-17

Jacobs SC, Berg SI, Lawson RK (1980) Synchrones bilateral renal cell carcinoma: total surgical excision. Cancer 46:2341-2345

Morgan WR, Zincke H (1990) Progression and survival after renal-conserving surgery for renal cell carcinoma; experience in 104 patients and extended follow-up. J Urol 144:852-857

Novick AC, Jackson CL, Straffon RA (1990) The role of renal autotransplantation in complex urological reconstruction. J. Urol 143(3):452-457

Pettersson S, Brynger H, Johansson S, Nilson AE (1979) Extracorporeal surgery and autotransplantation for carcinoma of the pelvis and ureter. Scand J Urol Nephrol 13:89-93

Pettersson S, Aamot P, Brynger H, Johansson S, Nilson AE, Ranch T (1981) Extracorporeal renal surgery, autotransplantation, and calicovesicostomy for renal pelvic and ureteric tumours. Scand J Urol Nephrol [Suppl] 60:33-35

Rhame RC (1973) Application of renal autotransplantation to the treatment of simultaneous bilateral ureteral tumours. Brit J Urol 45:388-390

Rohl L, Dreikorn K, Heering H (1979) Organerthaltende Chirurgie bei der Behandlung von Nierentumoren im Solitärnieren und doppelseitigen Nierentumoren. Helv Chir Acta 46(3):309-313

Scott R (1966) Tumour removal attempt on work-bench. Trans Am Assoc Genitourin Surg 58:111-113

Smith RB, de Kernion JB, Ehrlich RM, Skinner DG, Kaufman JJ (1984) Bilateral renal cell carcinoma and renal cell carcinoma in the solitary kidney. J Urol 132:450- 454

Stormont TJ, Bilhartz DL, Zincke H (1992) Pitfalls of "bench surgery" and autotransplantion for renal cell carcinoma. Mayo Clinic Proc 67(7):621-628

Topley M, Novick AC, Montie JE (1984) Long-term results following partial nephrectomy for localized renal adenocarcinoma. J Urol 131:1050-1052

Wickham JEA (1975) Conservative renal surgery for adenocarcinoma. The place of bench surgery. Brit J Urol 47:25-36

Zincke H, Engen DE, Henning KM, McDonald MW (1985) Treatment of renal cell carcinoma by in situ partial nephrectomy and extracorporeal operation with autotransplantation. Mayo Clin Proc 60:651-662

Simultaneous Aortic Reconstruction and Renal Autotransplantation

Inge B. Brekke, Ole Øyen, Robert Innes, and Audun Flatmark

10.1
Introduction

Renal revascularization is part of the procedure when repairing pararenal abdominal aortic aneurysms (AAAs). This combined approach may also be indicated for juxtarenal AAA or when infrarenal aortic aneurysmal or occlusive disease coexists with renal artery stenosis (RAS).

Juxtarenal AAAs (Bergan and Trippel 1963; Crawford et al. 1986) are defined as aneurysms that involve the infrarenal abdominal aorta adjacent to or including the lower margin of renal artery origin (Fig. 10.1A). Pararenal aneurysms involve the orifice of at least one renal artery (Fig. 10.1B) and may extend proximal to include the visceral vessels.

These constellations often represent a considerable therapeutic challenge, including problems with regard to surgical exposure and ischemic organ damage. Suprarenal aortic clamping, required for repair of juxtarenal and pararenal aneurysms, involves risk of postoperative renal insufficiency secondary to renal ischemia/reperfusion injury. The addition of in situ renal artery surgery prolongs the renal ischemia period and thus significantly increases the risk of renal damage (Nypaver et al. 1993; Tarazi et al. 1987).

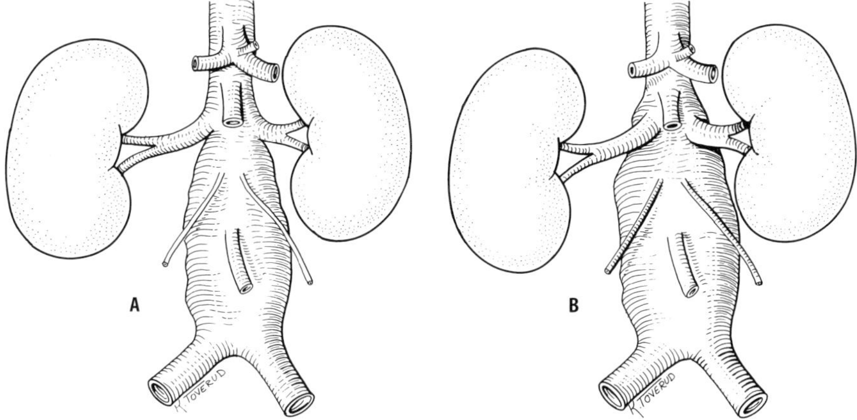

Fig. 10.1A,B. Juxta- (A) and pararenal (B) abdominal aortic aneurysms

In series published during the 1960s and 1970s, the addition of renal artery surgery to aortic reconstruction was associated with a significant mortality rate (10%-31%; DeBakey et al. 1964; Sanger et al. 1967; Gomes and Bernatz 1970; Ernst et al. 1973; Foster et al. 1975). The combined procedure was therefore recommended only for very restrictive indications. The surgical mortality of the combined procedure has largely been reduced in most subsequent series (Shahian et al. 1980; Stewart et al. 1985; Huffman and Johnson 1988; Branchereau et al. 1992), while others still report a twofold or threefold increase in mortality compared with aortic repair alone (Dean et al. 1984; Tarazi et al. 1987; Piquet et al. 1988).

On the whole, however, the results in terms of patient survival have improved considerably over the last two decades, mainly thanks to better understanding of risk factors and improved perioperative hemodynamic monitoring (Qvarfordt et al. 1986; Hollier and Moore 1990; Stenseth 1990). However, postoperative renal insufficiency caused by ischemia-induced tubular necrosis is still a prominent complication occurring in 23% or more of all cases in series involving surgery of the upper abdominal aorta (Crawford et al. 1986; Qvarfordt et al. 1986; Breckwoldt et al. 1992). Renal failure is supposed to be the most common factor in early postoperative death. In the overwhelming majority of these reports the renal revascularization procedure has been performed by various in situ bypass techniques, and renal clamp time has been shown to be a statistically significant predictor of early postoperative renal failure (Crawford et al. 1986). Several methods have been advocated to minimize renal complications. These include renal artery perfusion with various perfusates, such as oxygenated blood (Ochsner et al. 1984) or, more commonly, saline solutions (Allen et al. 1993; Green et al. 1989; Svensson et al. 1989). Nevertheless, postoperative renal insufficiency continues to be a major concern in these patients. Therefore, renal autotransplantation, with extracorporeal cold renal storage and retransplantation subsequent to aortic replacement represents an interesting alternative to in situ techniques for renal artery reconstruction and revascularization.

10.2
Prevalence of Aortorenal Disease

10.2.1
Juxta- and Pararenal Aortic Aneurysms

Juxtarenal (Fig. 10.1A) and pararenal AAAs (Fig. 10.1B) are being diagnosed with increasing frequency. This reflects the increasing average age of the general population, as well as improved diagnostic techniques, such as biplane aortography, computed tomography (Gomes and Choyke 1987), and magnetic resonance imaging (see Chap. 2).

The reported incidence of juxta- or pararenal AAA varies from 2% to 20% of AAAs (Crawford et al. 1986; Hollier and Moore 1990; Qvarfordt et al. 1986; Poulias et al. 1992).

In a 5-year retrospective review of 174 abdominal aortic aneurysmectomies performed, Taylor et al. (1994) found that 15.5% involved the juxtarenal aorta, while Lacroix et al. (1994) reported 25 cases or 5.8% out of 429 abdominal aneurysms. In a multicenter, nationwide prospective study of 666 nonruptured AAAs, 6.8% of repairs required clamping above the renal arteries (Johnston and Scobie 1988). This disparity probably reflects variations in preoperative work-up as well as differences in level of care, referral patterns, and classification methods, with the actual incidence probably being higher than reported.

10.2.2
Coexistent Aortic and Renal Artery Disease

The coexistence of an infrarenal aortic aneurysm or occlusive disease and RAS (Fig. 10.2) is likewise increasingly observed. In recent publications renal artery lesions are encountered in 20%-50% of patients with infrarenal aortic pathology (Brewster et al. 1975; Baur et al. 1978; Olin et al. 1990).

However, in a published review (Branchereau et al. 1992), the percentage of combined aortic and renal artery reconstruction is considerably lower, and in most series below 10%. In a series of more than 1000 aortic reconstructions, renal revascularization was performed in 3.2% only (Shahian et al. 1980), whereas Dean et al. (1984) reported a rate of 18.5%.

The majority of significant renal artery stenoses seen today will be treated primarily with percutaneous transluminal renal angioplasty (PTRA). In contrast to stenoses caused by fibromuscular disease, however, the atherosclerotic stenoses have a very high recurrence rate (Weibull et al. 1993), necessitating surgical reconstruction in several patients.

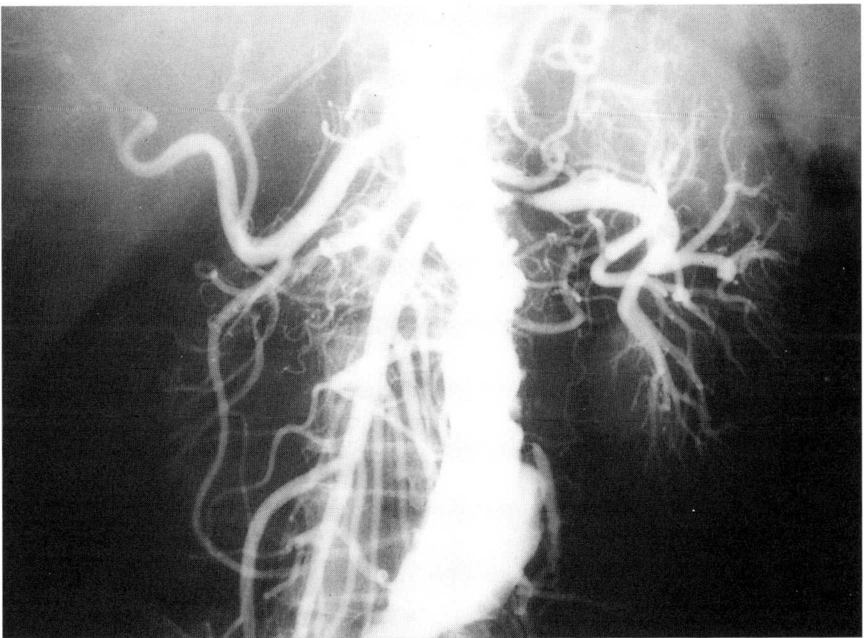

Fig. 10.2. Severe atherosclerosis of the infrarenal abdominal aorta and the left renal artery

10.3
Indications for a Combined Procedure

Surgical intervention for aortorenal disease may be mandatory to prevent lower limb gangrene, rupture of the AAA, to salvage one or both kidneys, or to treat severe hypertension when PTRA has failed.

Emergency intervention with simultaneous repair of the abdominal aorta and renal artery may be required in patients with aortorenal disease complicated by acute renal artery occlusion or ruptured AAA (Versteegh 1977; MacMillan et al. 1988; Ross et al. 1989; Flatmark et al. 1989), as in eight of the 83 patients in our own series.

In elective treatment, the increased risk associated with the combined aortic and renal artery reconstruction in the often elderly patient must be weighed against the severity of symptoms and the dubious prognosis of the untreated aortic and renal artery disease diagnosed. Factors such as the severity of renovascular hypertension, compromised renal function, imminent lower extremity gangrene, estimated risk of renal artery occlusion, or aneurysm rupture must all be taken into account (Atnip et al. 1990; Hallett et al. 1992; Brothers et al. 1995). The decision to operate or not will depend on a thorough evaluation of these factors as well as age and general condition of the patient.

In patients with infrarenal aortic aneurysms or occlusive disease and RAS, the RAS may be treated separately by PTRA. The indication for simultaneous repair in these patients is usually manifest when a significant RAS has proven to be unmanageable by PTRA.

It should also be kept in mind that asymptomatic or minimally symptomatic RAS can progress to renal artery occlusion. Prophylactic revascularization of these lesions at the time of aortic surgery may be indicated to ensure kidney function (Pohl and Novick 1985; Tollefson and Ernst 1991).

10.4
Preoperative Assessment

Accurate preoperative assessment of the aortic pathology and renal artery involvement, accessory renal arteries, and other vascular abnormalities is of importance when planning surgical strategy. Ultrasonography is valuable in diagnosing AAA, but not reliable in determining renal artery involvement or evaluating the thoracic aorta. Conventional CT demonstrates the renal artery origins in most cases (Gomes and Choyke 1987). However, we believe that biplane aortography is indicated in all patients with a large AAA (see Chap. 2). The preoperative evaluation should include visualization of the complete aorta, including the aortic arch and the iliac arteries.

When renal artery involvement is diagnosed or suspected, radionuclide renal scanning is performed to determine the function of each kidney separately (see Chap. 3). If the function of one kidney is reduced to, let us say, 10%-15% or less of normal, while the contralateral kidney has a near to normal function, removal of the poorly functioning kidney should be planned as part of the operation.

Several factors have been identified that increase the risk of death of patients undergoing surgery for extensive aortic aneurysms, the most important being ischemic heart disease, renal dysfunction, and chronic obstructive airway disease (Crawford et al. 1986; Hallett et al. 1992; Brothers et al. 1995). Several studies have shown a high prevalence of coronary artery disease (CAD) among patients with combined renal and peripheral vascular disease, suggesting RAS to be an independent marker for CAD (Hallett et al. 1992; Valentine et al. 1993). Consequently, about 50% of the perioperative morbidity and mortality of simultaneous aortic and renal artery surgery has been ascribed to CAD (Cunningham 1989; Valentine et al. 1993).

Thus, advanced RAS in a patient with peripheral vascular disease is a strong indication for meticulous preoperative cardiac evaluation, including stress electrocardiograph and thallium scanning or coronary angiography. This evaluation should be performed routinely in all these patients, as a high percentage have serious coronary heart disease without symptoms (Hertzer et al. 1984). When coronary revascularization is indicated, this should be given priority before aortorenal revascularization.

There are well-known changes in pulmonary physiology associated with major abdominal surgery per- and postoperatively. Pulmonary function should therefore be investigated when appropriate, and measures taken to optimize pulmonary function prior to surgery.

In the 22-year period from 1973 to 1995, 83 patients were treated with simultaneous aortic and renal artery reconstruction at the National Hospital in Oslo. Preoperative patient data are given in Table 10.1. Aortic aneurysm was present in 45 of the patients, while atherosclerotic stenosis of renal artery and aorta was the predominant finding in 38. The aortic aneurysm was symptomatic in 20 patients (44%), including eight who were treated as an emergency for rupture or impending rupture. Thirty-one of the patients, or almost 40%, had symptomatic coronary heart disease. Preoperative cardiovascular evaluation of the patients, to grade the severity of disease or detect asymptomatic coronary disease, was routinely performed during the last few years only.

Table 10.1. Preoperative data on 83 patients treated with simultaneous aortic and renal artery reconstruction

Mean age (range)	Gender M/F	Aortic aneurysm (n)	Aortic stenosis (n)	Hyper-tension[a] (n)	Coronary disease[b] (n)	Renal in-sufficiency[c] (n)
58 (19-77)	54/29	45	38	70	31	44

[a] Medically treated hypertension
[b] Symptomatic coronary heart disease
[c] No. of patients with creatinine above 130 µmol/l

10.5
Surgery

10.5.1
Peroperative Management

Simultaneous aortic reconstruction and renal revascularization require close cooperation between surgeons and experienced anesthesiologists. All patients should be monitored with electrocardiograph, invasive radial artery pressure, central venous pressure, pulse oximetry and multi-gas analysis (Stenseth 1990). Although spinal cord damage has been reported after abdominal aortic clamping (Szilagyi et al. 1978), this is extremely rare and prophylactic measures such as cerebrospinal fluid drainage are not routinely performed in subdiaphragmatic aortic clamping. General anesthesia should be supplemented by epidural analgesia unless there are specific contraindications such as coagulopathy. This is despite the fact that epidural anesthesia may itself very occasionally cause serious neurological sequels or receive the blame for spinal cord injury actually associated with ischemia due to the surgery (Breivik 1995).

Peroperative autotransfusion reduces the need for homologous blood transfusion. Antibiotic prophylaxis is started at induction of anesthesia. Mannitol and diuretics are given before renal artery clamping (see Chap. 4).

10.5.2
Aortic Replacement and Renal Autotransplantation

While many juxtarenal AAAs may be treated by the incorporation of the renal artery orifices into the suture line of the proximal anastomosis (Crawford et al. 1986), renal artery reconstruction is part of the surgical procedure during repair of the pararenal AAA. In most cases of juxta- as well as pararenal AAAs, however, we feel that it is safer to remove the kidneys and autotransplant them in conjunction with the aortic replacement. In centers experienced in renal transplantation, simultaneous aortic replacement and renal autotransplantation offer a safe alternative to the in situ bypass procedures preferred by many vascular surgeons.

Removing the kidney(s) before handling the aorta prevents microembolization to the renal parenchyma (trash kidney), and extracorporeal cold storage preserves renal function. At least in patients with a single functioning kidney, this is probably the procedure which best ensures a nonazotemic outcome.

The right tributaries of the aorta, the right renal artery, and the common iliac artery are best approached by a transperitoneal route. Our standard approach to the abdominal aorta is through a midline laparotomy with the patient supine. Examination of the intraperitoneal organs, which is the first stage of the operation, will reveal pathological processes, such as infectious diseases or cancer, which may contraindicate the vascular procedure. As the next step, depending on whether one or both kidneys are affected, uni- or bilateral nephrectomy is performed according to the technique described in Chap. 4. The kidney(s) are placed in a basin with iced Ringer Acetate, perfused with Euro Collins solution, and kept cooled until retransplanted (see Chaps. 4 and 5).

Various maneuvers may be applied in order to control the cranial end of a pararenal aneurysm. Mobilization of the duodenum facilitates approach to the origin of the superior mesenteric artery. The supraceliac part of the aorta may be reached from the right side through the crux of the diaphragm, or exposure of the entire abdominal aorta is achieved from the left by medial mobilization of the left colon, the spleen, and the pancreas.

Depending on the local condition of the aortic wall, the aorta may be clamped (a) below the superior mesenteric artery (SMA), (b) between the SMA and celiac artery, or (c) above the celiac artery. There has been some concern about the changes in cardiac afterload associated with supraceliac aortic cross-clamping. The simplicity of dissection in this area required for supraceliac placement of the clamp, however, is claimed to reduce the risk of iatrogenic complications and should therefore probably be practiced more liberally (Nypaver et al. 1993).

The diseased aorta is replaced by a synthetic graft while a second team of surgeons perform the required bench surgery on the kidney(s) (see Chap. 7).

After completion of the aortic replacement, the kidney(s) are transplanted to the pelvic region, where the renal artery is anastomosed to the aortic graft or to the internal or external iliac artery as described in Chap. 5 and shown in Figs. 10.3 and 10.4. A ureteroneocystostomy is constructed after completion of the vascular anastomoses and renal revascularization.

10.6
Postoperative Care and Evaluation

Maintenance of cardiovascular stability is the main objective in the immediate postoperative course. Optimal renal function is preserved by maintaining adequate intravascular volume and blood pressure. The use of epidural anesthesia during the first postoperative days decreases the need for opiates and thus the incidence of cardiopulmonary morbidity (Breivik 1995).

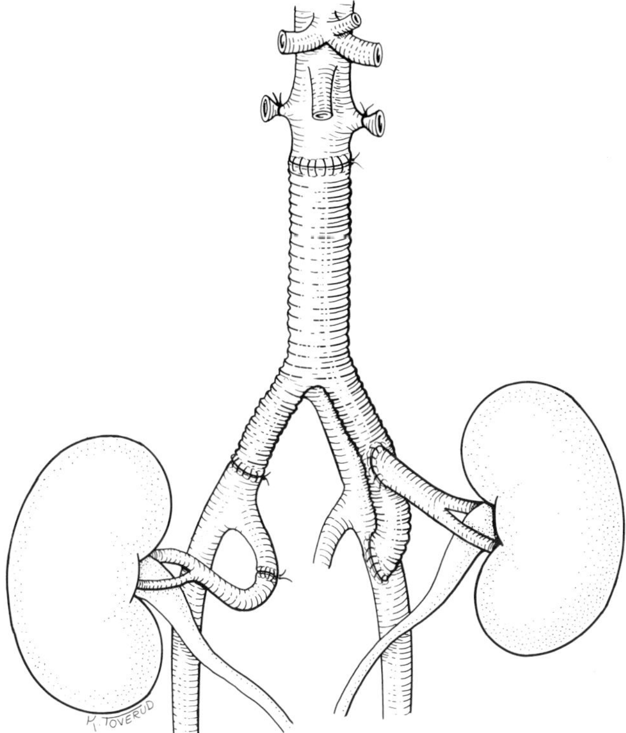

Fig. 10.3. Aorto-biiliac bypass and bilateral renal autotransplantation with renal artery anastomosis to the aortic prosthesis on the left side, and to the internal iliac artery on the right side

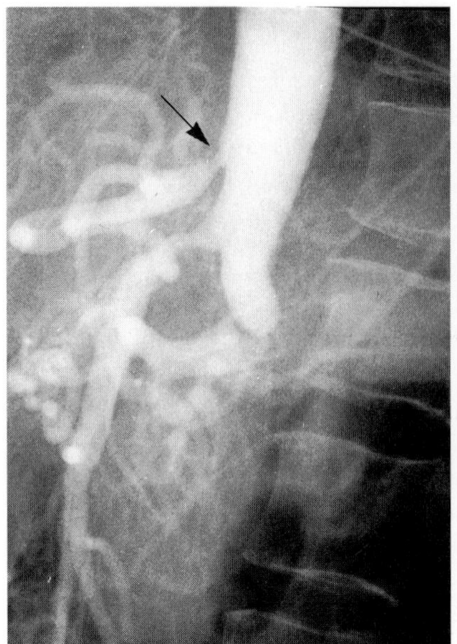

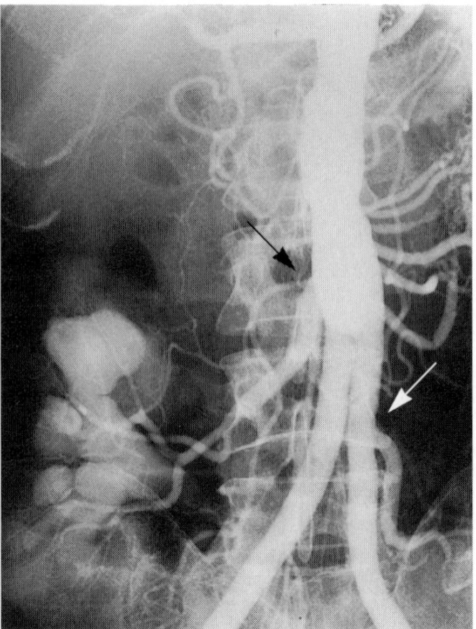

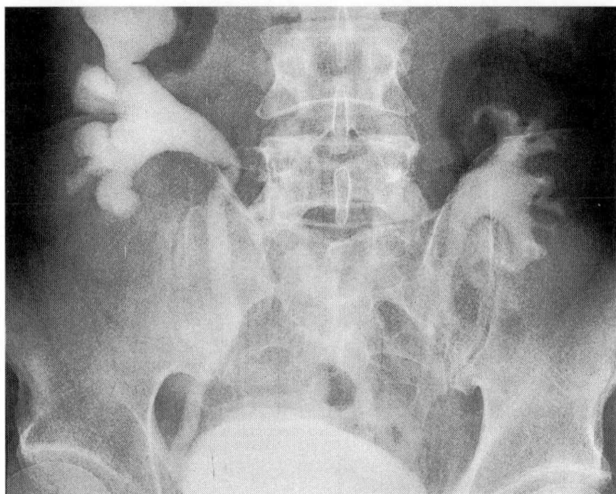

Fig. 10.4 A-C. Stenosis of the right renal artery ($\rightarrow$), occluded left renal artery and abdominal aorta (A), treated by aortic replacement and bilateral renal autotransplantation. Both renal arteries anastomosed to the aortic prosthesis ($\rightarrow$) (B). Good function in both autotransplants and unrestricted ureteral passage demonstrated by urography (C)

Autotransplant function is monitored by urinary output and serum creatinine. Graft circulation is investigated by duplex ultrasonography, and arteriography is performed only when serious vascular complications are suspected. Ureteral obstruction is ruled out by ultrasound examinations and excretion urography (Fig. 10.4C). The function of each kidney is estimated separately by isotope radionuclide scans.

The patient is readmitted 3 months after surgery, and later annually, for a general follow-up examination, including renal function tests, duplex ultrasonography, and radionuclide renal scans.

10.7
Results

10.7.1
Perioperative Morbidity and Mortality

As already mentioned, several reports have pointed out that simultaneous aortic and renal revascularization is associated with a considerable increase in mortality rate compared with aortic repair alone. Crawford et al. (1986) concluded that renal failure was the most common complication and the most common factor in the cause of early death, following surgery on juxtarenal aortic aneurysms keeping the kidneys in situ. Postoperative renal failure is closely related to renal artery clamp time and the presence of renal artery occlusive disease. In most reports, the rate of postoperative renal insufficiency varies between 15% and 26% (Eriksson et al. 1988). When additional surgery is performed on the renal arteries, renal failure is reported to occur in 15%-61% of the cases (Crawford et al. 1986; Qvarfordt et al. 1986; Eriksson et al. 1988).

Reported surgical mortality for juxtarenal aneurysmectomy with or without simultaneous renal artery repair ranges from 1.3% to 31% (Crawford et al. 1986; Qvarfordt et al. 1986; Eriksson et al. 1988; Brothers et al. 1995). This probably reflects different selection criteria. In the series presented by Crawford et al. (1986), the early death rate of patients with associated renal artery stenosis was 20%, and Eriksson et al. (1988) found that patients with bilateral renal artery disease had twice the early mortality rate of patients with unilateral lesions.

In our series of 83 combined procedures performed since 1973, 44 had impaired renal function preoperatively (Tables 10.1, 10.2). Bilateral renal artery revascularization was performed in 21 patients. Seventeen patients (20%) died postoperatively. The most frequent cause of death was myocardial infarction (six patients), followed by sepsis and multiorgan failure (five patients). All but one of these deaths occurred in patients treated before 1990.

Table 10.2. Surgical details in 83 patients treated with simultaneous aortic and renal artery reconstruction

Unilat. autotx L/R	Bilateral autotx n	Nephrectomy* L/R	Renal artery to prosthesis
32/30	21	13/10	46

* Concomitant removal of a contralateral, non-functioning or marginally functioning kidney

10.7.2
Effect on Blood Pressure and Renal Function

Renal autotransplantation for RVH has been reported to normalize or improve blood pressure in 90%-100% of patients treated (Merguerian et al. 1990; Novick 1991; Brekke et al. 1992) and preserve or improve renal function in 85%-100% (Lacombe 1989; Brekke et al. 1992; Murray et al. 1994). These results are superior to the 60%-80% improvement in RVH, reportedly achieved by in situ techniques (Mattila et al. 1985; Stewart et al. 1985; Qvarfordt et al. 1986).

While 84% of the patients in our series were hypertensive before surgery, defined as using one or more antihypertensive drugs, blood pressure was normalized or improved in 84% of the long-term surviving, previously hypertensive patients. In these patients, surgery was associated with a reduction in the mean number of antihypertensive drugs taken per patient, from 3.5 to 1.1 (Table 10.3).

Table 10.3. Results of simultaneous aortic and renal artery reconstruction. Mean values and number of patients with claudication, 3-12 months after surgery

	Blood pressure[a] (no. of drugs)	Creatinine (μmol/l)	ERPF[b] (%)	Claudication (no. of patients)
Preoperative	3.5	202	59.8	39
Postoperative	1.1	182	60.1	1

[a] Mean number of antihypertensive drugs used
[b] Effective renal plasma flow. Percentage of estimated normal

Renal function was preserved in all 66 long-term survivors. Functional improvement (creatinine reduction of more than 30 μmol/l) was observed in 18 of these, reduction (creatinine increase of more than 30 μmol/l) in 15, while renal function remained unchanged in 33 patients.

10.8
Summary

Patients with renovascular disease concomitant with aneurysm or atherosclerotic occlusive disease of the abdominal aorta represent a considerable therapeutic challenge. The results of simultaneous aortic and renal artery reconstruction depend not only on surgical skills, but to a great extent on the often preexisting risk factors in these patients, such as high patient age, diffuse atherosclerotic disease, impaired renal function, and cardiopulmonary disease. To preoperatively optimize the state of the patient, and particularly the cardiopulmonary state, is therefore of outmost importance.

When the decision has been made in favor of surgical reconstruction, the surgeon is faced with a complex task requiring extensive experience in vascular surgery. In situ renal artery bypass procedures include aorto-, ileo-, spleno-, and hepatorenal bypasses and are the most widely used revascularization techniques for renovascular disease. However, the impaired renal function often present in patients with aorto-renal disease implies reduced tolerance to renal ischemia. Furthermore, with an increased average age of the population, an increasing number of patients present with severe atherosclerotic disease including the pararenal aorta as well as the renal arteries (Libertino et al. 1988). This complicates procedures based on in situ bypass techniques, and the majority of reports on in situ renal revascularization state postoperative renal insufficiency to be a major problem. Placement of an aortic clamp near the origin of the renal arteries may cause fragmentation of atherosclerotic plaques, resulting in renal artery stenosis or embolization (Green et al. 1989). Surgical reintervention is often required in these patients (Stanley et al. 1985).

In selected patients, renal autotransplantation has been reported to be an excellent alternative to bypass techniques in the surgical treatment of renovascular hypertension, with normalization of blood pressure in the majority of patients treated (Sicard et al. 1988; Merguerian et al. 1990). Several authors have claimed that the results of autotransplantation are generally superior to conventional renal artery revascularization procedures (Dubernard et al. 1985; van Bockel et al. 1988).

Our own experience is based on 502 renal autotransplantations performed in 471 patients, of which 83 were treated with combined aortic replacement and revascularization of 104 kidneys. Based on this experience we recommend bench surgery and renal autotransplantation combined with aortic replacement as a valid alternative to in situ bypass techniques in the treatment of aortorenal disease. The concomitant autotransplantation of one or both kidneys surely implies an increased load on the patient, with increased operation time and extended dissection. The 20% postoperative mortality in our series reflects the high rate of risk factors present in our patients and underlines the importance of preoperative cardiovascular and pulmonary evaluation and treatment. This is further demonstrated by the significantly reduced lethal complication rate (8.3%) since 1989, when the preoperative evaluation of the patients was intensified.

In centers familiar with renal transplantation, bench surgery ensures optimal preservation of renal function and the best prospects for blood pressure normalization or improvement. The benefits of preserving renal function and ameliorating hypertension are substantial, and the surgical risk should be weighed against the hazards of long-term dialysis.

References

Allen BT, Anderson CB, Rubin BG, Flye MW, Baumann DS, Sicard GA (1993) Preservation of renal function in juxtarenal and suprarenal abdominal aortic aneurysm repair. J Vasc Surg 17(5):948-958

Atnip RG, Neumyer MM, Healy DA, Thiele BL (1990) Combined aortic and visceral arterial reconstruction: risks and results. J Vasc Surg 12(6):705-714

Baur GM, Porter JM, Eidemiller LR, Rosch J, Keller F (1978) The role of arteriography in abdominal aortic aneurysm. Am J Surg 136(2):184-189

Bergan JJ, Trippel OH (1963) Management of juxtarenal aortic occlusions. Arch Surg 87:230-238

Branchereau A, Espinoza H, Magnan PE, Rosset E, Castro M (1992) Simultaneous reconstruction of infrarenal abdominal aorta and renal arteries (review). Ann Vasc Surg 6(3):232-238

Breckwoldt WL, Mackey WC, Belkin M, O'Donnell TJ (1992) The effect of suprarenal cross-clamping on abdominal aortic aneurysm repair. Arch Surg 127(5):520-524

Breivik H (1995) Benefits, risks and economics of post-operative pain management programmes. Baillieres Clin Anaesth 9:403-422

Brekke IB, Sodal G, Jakobsen A, Bentdal O, Pfeffer P, Albrechtsen D, Flatmark A (1992) Fibro-muscular renal artery disease treated by extracorporeal vascular reconstruction and renal autotransplantation: short- and long-term results. Eur J Vasc Surg 6(5):471-476

Brewster DC, Retana A, Waltman AC, Darling RC (1975) Angiography in the management of aneurysms of the abdominal aorta. Its value and safety. N Engl J Med 292(16):822-825

Brothers TE, Elliott BM, Robison JG, Rajagopalan PR (1995) Stratification of mortality risk for renal artery surgery. Am Surg 61(1):45-51

Crawford ES, Beckett WC, Greer MS (1986) Juxtarenal infrarenal abdominal aortic aneurysm. Special diagnostic and therapeutic considerations. Ann Surg 203(6):661-670

Cunningham AJ (1989) Anaesthesia for abdominal aortic surgery-a review (Part II) (review). Can J Anaesth 36(5):568-577

Dean RH, Keyser J, Dupont WD, Nadeau JH, Meacham PW (1984) Aortic and renal vascular disease. Factors affecting the value of combined procedures. Ann Surg 200(3):336-344

DeBakey ME, Morris GC Jr, Morgan RO (1964) Lesions of the renal artery: surgical technique and results. Am J Surg 107:84-96

Dubernard JM, Martin X, Gelet A, Mongin D, Canton F, Tabib A (1985) Renal autotransplantation versus bypass techniques for renovascular hypertension. Surgery 97(5):529-534

Eriksson I, Bowald S, Karacagil S (1988) Surgical treatment of pararenal abdominal aortic aneurysms. Int Angiol 7(1):7-13

Ernst CB, Stanley JC, Marshall FF, Fry WJ (1973) Renal revascularization for arteriosclerotic renovascular hypertension: prognostic implications of focal renal arterial vs. overt generalized arteriosclerosis. Surgery 73(6):859-867

Flatmark A, Albrechtsen D, Sodal G, Bondevik H, Jakobsen AJ, Brekke IB (1989) Renal autotransplantation. World J Surg 13(2):206-209

Foster JH, Maxwell MH, Franklin SS, Bleifer KH, Trippel OH, Julian OC, DeCamp PT, Varady PT (1975) Renovascular occlusive disease. Results of operative treatment. JAMA 231(10):1043-1048

Gomes MM, Bernatz PE (1970) Aorto-iliac occlusive disease. Extension cephalad to origin of renal arteries, with surgical considerations and results. Arch Surg 101(2):161-166

Gomes MN, Choyke PL (1987) Improved identification of renal arteries in patients with aortic aneurysms by means of high-resolution computed tomography. J Vasc Surg 6(3):262-268

Green RM, Ricotta JJ, Ouriel K, DeWeese JA (1989) Results of supraceliac aortic clamping in the difficult elective resection of infrarenal abdominal aortic aneurysm. J Vasc Surg 9:125-134

Hallett JJ, Schirger A, Bower TC, Cherry KJ, Gloviczki P, Pairolero PC (1992) The current role of surgical revascularization for combined renovascular hypertension and renal insufficiency (review). Int Angiol 11(1):64-68

Hertzer NR, Beven EG, Young JR (1984) Coronary artery disease in peripheral vascular patients. A classification of 1000 coronary angiograms and results of surgical management. Ann Surg 199:223-233

Hollier LH, Moore WM (1990) Surgical management of juxtarenal and suprarenal aortic aneurysms. Acta Chir Scand Suppl 555(117):117-122

Huffman AD, Johnson RC (1988) Renal artery reconstruction: extended indications. South Med J 81(4):440-443

Johnston KW, Scobie TK (1988) Multicenter prospective study of nonruptured abdominal aortic aneurysms. I. Population and operative management. J Vasc Surg 7(1):69-81

Lacombe M (1989) Ex situ surgical repair of complex lesions of the renal artery (in French). Chirurgie 115(9):631-635

Lacroix H, Nevelsteen A, Dams A, Suy R (1994) Approach to aortic aneurysms including the renal arteries: retroperitoneal method (in French). J Mal Vasc 19:78-84

Libertino JA, Flam TA, Zinman LN, Ying CY, Breslin DJ, Swinton NJ, Phelps MJ, Tsapatsaris NP, Woods BO (1988) Changing concepts in surgical management of renovascular hypertension. Arch Intern Med 148(2):357-359

MacMillan RD, Uldall R, Lipton IH (1988) Simultaneous aortic and renal artery econstruction for acute arterial occlusion in solitary kidney. Urology 31(1):66-69

Mattila T, Harjola PT, Ketonen P, Varstela E, Hekali P (1985) Isolated renal artery and combined aortic and renal artery reconstruction for renovascular hypertension. Late results of surgical treatment. Ann Clin Res 17(1):19-23

Merguerian PA, McLorie GA, Balfe JW, Khoury AE, Churchill BM (1990) Renal autotransplantation in children: a successful treatment for renovascular hypertension. J Urol 144(6):1443-1445

Murray SP, Kent C, Salvatierra O, Stoney RJ (1994) Complex branch renovascular disease: management options and late results. J Vasc Surg 20(3):338-345

Novick AC (1991) Management of renovascular disease. A surgical perspective (review). Circulation 83[suppl I]:1167-1171

Nypaver TJ, Shepard AD, Reddy DJ, Elliott JJ, Smith RF, Ernst CB (1993) Repair of pararenal abdominal aortic aneurysms. An analysis of operative management. Arch Surg 128(7):803-811

Ochsner JL, Mills NL, Gardner PA (1984) A technique for renal preservation during suprarenal abdominal aortic operations. Surg Gynecol Obstet 159(4):388-390

Olin JW, Melia M, Young JR, Graor RA, Risius B (1990) Prevalence of atherosclerotic renal artery stenosis in patients with atherosclerosis elsewhere. Am J Med 88(1N):46N-51N

Piquet P, Ocana J, Verdon E, Tournigand P, Mercier C (1988) Atherosclerotic lesions of the aorta and renal arteries: results of simultaneous surgical treatment. Ann Vasc Surg 2(4):319-325

Pohl MA, Novick AC (1985) Natural history of atherosclerotic and fibrous renal artery disease: clinical implications (review). Am J Kidney Dis 5(4):A120-A130

Poulias GE, Doundoulakis N, Skoutas B, Prombonas E, Haddad H, Papaioannou K, Lymberiadis D, Savopoulos G (1992) Juxtarenal abdominal aneurysmectomy. J Cardiovasc Surg (Torino) 33(3):324-330

Qvarfordt PG, Stoney RJ, Reilly LM, Skioldebrand CG, Goldstone J, Ehrenfeld WK (1986) Management of pararenal aneurysms of the abdominal aorta. J Vasc Surg 3(1):84-93

Ross WB, Markham NI, Salaman JR (1989) Autotransplantation for renovascular hypertension with complete renal artery occlusion. Ann R Coll Surg Engl 71(4):233-235

Sanger PW, Daugherty HK, Robicsek F, Gallucci V (1967) Aorticorenal disease. A surgical entity. Ann Thorac Surg 3(3):195-203

Shahian DM, Najafi H, Javid H, Hunter JA, Goldin MD, Monson DO (1980) Simultaneous aortic and renal artery reconstruction. Arch Surg 115(12):1491-1497

Sicard GA, Valentin LI, Freeman MB, Allen BT, Anderson CB (1988) Renal autotransplantation: an alternative to standard renal revascularization procedures. Surgery 104(4):624-630

Stanley JC, Whitehouse WJ, Zelenock GB, Graham LM, Cronenwett JL, Lindenauer SM (1985) Reoperation for complications of renal artery reconstructive surgery undertaken for treatment of renovascular hypertension. J Vasc Surg 2(1):133-144

Stenseth R (1990) Advances in anaesthesiological management of aortic surgery. Acta Chir Scand Suppl 555(123):123-128

Stewart MT, Smith R , Fulenwider JT, Perdue GD, Wells JO (1985) Concomitant renal revascularization in patients undergoing aortic surgery. J Vasc Surg 2(3):400-405

Svensson LG, Coselli JS, Safi HJ, Hess KR, Crawford ES (1989) Appraisal of adjuncts to prevent acute renal failure after surgery on the thoracic or thoracoabdominal aorta. J Vasc Surg 10(3):230-239

Szilagyi DE, Hageman JH, Smith RF, Elliott JP (1978) Spinal cord damage in surgery of the abdominal aorta. Surgery 83(1):38-56

Tarazi RY, Hertzer NR, Beven EG, O'Hara PJ, Anton GE, Krajewski LP (1987) Simultaneous aortic reconstruction and renal revascularization: risk factors and late results in eighty-nine patients. J Vasc Surg 5(5):707-714

Taylor SM, Mills JL, Fujitani RM (1994) The juxtarenal abdominal aortic aneurysm. A more common problem than previously realized? Arch Surg 129(7):734-737

Tollefson DF, Ernst CB (1991) Natural history of atherosclerotic renal artery stenosis associated with aortic disease. J Vasc Surg 14(3):327-331

Valentine RJ, Clagett GP, Miller GL, Myers SI, Martin JD, Chervu A (1993) The coronary risk of unsuspected renal artery stenosis. J Vasc Surg 18(3):433-439

van Bockel JH, van Schilfgaarde R, Overbosch EH, Felthuis W, Terpstra JL (1988) The influence of the surgical technique upon the short term and long term anatomic results in reconstructive operation for renovascular hypertension. Surg Gynecol Obstet 166(5):402-408

Versteegh PM (1977) Ruptured aneurysm of the abdominal aorta with kidney autografting. Arch Chir Neerl 29(1):63-67

Weibull H, Bergqvist D, Bergentz SE, Jonsson K, Hulthen L, Manhem P (1993) Percutaneous transluminal renal angioplasty versus surgical reconstruction of atherosclerotic renal artery stenosis: a prospective randomized study. J Vasc Surg 18(5):841-850

Management of Ureteral Defects by Renal Autotransplantation

Øystein H. Bentdal and Gunnar Sødal

11.1
Introduction

The management of ureteral defects by renal autotransplantation was first reported by Hardy in 1963, when he described the application of this technique in a patient with severe ureteral injury (Hardy 1963). Renal autotransplantation has since become an established procedure in the treatment of various urological disorders. Some authors have suggested ureteral injury, defect, or disorder to be a main indication for renal autotransplantation (Stewart et al. 1977; Novick et al. 1981; Rembrink et al. 1993). Rembrink et al. (1993) reported excellent results with this technique in the treatment of retroperitoneal fibrosis affecting the ureters, and renal autotransplantation has been shown to represent a valid therapeutic option in patients requiring replacement of all or a major portion of the ureter (Novick et al. 1990).

11.2
Alternative Surgical Techniques

Various surgical techniques have been developed to reestablish continuity between the kidney and urinary bladder and thus salvage kidney function in patients with a diseased or damaged ureter. The afflicted ureteral segment may be excised and the end of the remaining ureter reimplanted into the bladder or attached to the renal pelvis, depending on what part of the ureter is removed. If enough ureter is left, a reattachment can be performed without further manipulation. If a somewhat larger part of the ureter is removed, an anastomosis between the ureter and bladder may still be possible by mobilizing the bladder with a psoas hitch technique, or by making a tube of bladder wall as in the Boari flap technique, or by bringing the distal end of the ureter across to the contralateral ureter for a transureteroureteric anastomosis (Lieskovsky and Skinner 1986; Blandy et al. 1996; Ehrlich and Skinner 1975).

When the extent of ureteral damage is such that continuity between the kidney and urinary bladder cannot be reestablished by these techniques, the ureter may be replaced by a segment of ileum or the kidney may be autotransplanted to the pelvic region. In these cases we have given preference to renal autotransplantation.

11.3
Own Experience

Since 1976 we have performed renal autotransplantation for ureteral defects in 13 patients, 9 females and 4 males, aged 13 to 71 years (mean 46). Six of the patients had a single kidney. The indications for surgical treatment were iatrogenic ureteral defects in eight patients and stricture of the ureter in five (Table 11.1). The ureteral stricture was caused by irradiation in three patients treated for carcinoma of the uterus and by retroperitoneal fibrosis in two patients. The retroperitoneal fibrosis was caused by systemic lupus erythomatosus in one patient and was secondary to aortic graft implantation in the other. Renal autotransplantation was performed according to the surgical technique described in Chap. 5. When total ureteral resection was indicated, a pyelocystostomy was made as described in Chap. 8.

Table 11.1. Causes of ureteral disorders, giving indication for renal autotransplantation in 13 patients

Ureteral defects following surgery for

Nephrolithiasis	3
Vesicoureteral reflux	2
Hydronephrosis	1
Sigmoiditis	1
Aortoiliac atherosclerosis	1

Ureteral stricture caused by

Irradiation injury	3
Retroperitoneal fibrosis	2

Figure 11.1A illustrates a strictured distal ureter in a 19-year-old boy with a single kidney. A previously performed bilateral ureteroneocystostomy was followed by bilateral distal ureteral stricture. Subsequently, a nonfunctioning right kidney was removed. The remaining left kidney was autotransplanted to the right iliac region. The strictured segment of the ureter was excised and a ureteroneocystostomy performed. Pyelography of the autotransplant 3 months later shows a marked regression of hydronephrosis (Fig. 11.1B).

11.4
Results

Two autotransplanted kidneys were lost postoperatively. Graft loss was caused by renal artery occlusion in one patient who preoperatively had received multiple series of radiation treatment of the pelvic region for carcinoma of the uterus. The other graft loss occurred in a patient who had gone through multiple operations for nephrolithiasis before autotransplantation. Technical difficulties, due to rupture of a fragile renal vein resulted in renal vein thrombosis. Both patients had solitary kidneys and subsequently developed uremia. Both patients died 24 months after the autotransplantation due to septicemia. One of them received a kidney allograft 1 month before death, but the graft was lost in rejection.

Eleven patients were followed for 28-240 months (mean 127). The autotransplant function was unchanged during this time, with serum creatinine values in the range of 65-180 µmol/l (mean 111) at 24 months. Radionuclide split renal function tests were performed in all patients with two functioning kidneys, demonstrating well-preserved autotransplant function 24 months postoperatively, with unchanged effective renal plasma flow compared to preoperative values (150-300 ml/min; mean 220).

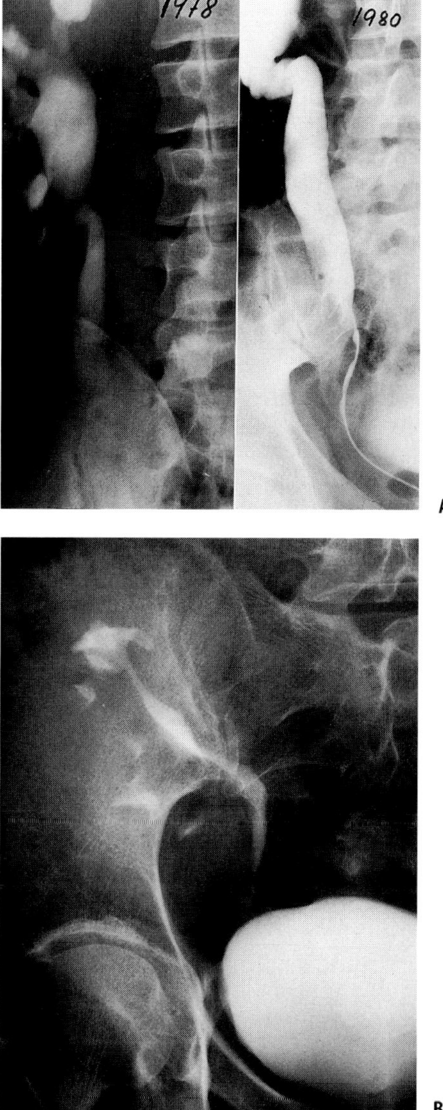

Fig. 11.1A,B. Pyelography of the right kidney before (A) and 3 months after autotransplantation and ureteroneocystostomy (B). A marked regression of hydronephrosis is demonstrated

11.5
Summary

Based on our own experience and on published series from other centers, it is concluded that renal autotransplantation grants good long-term results in the management of various ureteral defects and disorders. However, major abnormalities of renal or iliac vasculature may have implications on the safety of this procedure. Vascular complications related to preexisting disease may predispose for vascular thrombosis, as demonstrated in two of our patients.

All other patients in our series had excellent long-term kidney function and no surgical complications. Similar results were reported by Novick et al. (1990).

Surgeons not familiar with renal transplantation may prefer alternative surgical techniques. The most often used alternative for larger ureteral defects, the ileum interposition procedure, is reportedly often associated with severe and therapy-resistant urinary infections (Lieskovsky and Skinner 1986) and malfunction (Tanagho et al. 1975). Others have reported that ileal bridging of ureteral defects is a safe and useful procedure for properly selected patients (Fritzsche et al. 1975; Tveter and Goodwin 1982). The Boari-Ockerblad technique is probably the preferred and most reliable method for the management of distal ureteral defects (Bowsher et al. 1982; Blandy et al. 1991). However, we recommend that renal autotransplantation should be considered for all ureteral strictures or defects that are not restricted to the terminal ureter and thus not easily mastered by the more conventional procedures. In centers experienced in renal allotransplantation, this should be a very safe procedure, associated with a minimum of surgical complications.

References

Blandy J, Fowler C (1996) Iatrogenic injuries to the ureter. In: Blandy J and Fowler C (eds) Urology, 2nd edn. Blackwell Science, Oxford, pp 126-133

Bowsher WG, Shah PJR, Costello AJ, et al. (1982) A critical appraisal of the Boari flap. Br J Urol 54:682-685

Ehrlich RM, Skinner DG (1975) Complications of transureteroureterostomy. J Urol 113:467-470

Fritzsche P, Skinner DG, Goodwin WE, Craven JD, Cahill P (1975) Long-term radiographic changes of the kidney following the ileal ureter operation. J Urol 114:843-850

Hardy JD (1963) High ureteral injury: management by autotransplantation of the kidney. JAMA 184:97-101

Lieskovsky G, Skinner DG (1986) Use of intestinal segments in urinary tract. In: Cann C (ed) Campbell's urology, vol. 3, 5th edn. Saunders, Philadelphia, pp 2620-2638

Novick AC, Straffon RA, Stewart BH (1981) Experience with extracorporal renal operations and autotransplantation in the management of complicated urologic disorders. Surg Gynecol Obstet 153:10-18

Novick AC, Jackson CL, Straffon RA (1990) The role of renal autotransplantation in complex urological reconstruction. J Urol 143:452-457

Rembrink K, Niebel W, Behrendt H (1993) Autotransplantation of the kidney. Indications and results. Urologe A 32:151-155

Stewart BH, Banowsky LH, Hewitt CB, Straffon RA (1977) Renal autotransplantation: current perspectives. J Urol 118:363-368

Tanagho EA (1975) A case against incorporation of bowel segments into the closed urinary system. J Urol 114:843-850

Tveter KJ, Goodwin WE (1982) The use of ileum as substitute for the ureter. Curr Trend Urol 1:1

Subject Index

A
abdominal aortic aneurysms (AAA)
- infrarenal 125
- juxtarenal 125
- pararenal 125
acceleration
- index 26
- time 26
accessory arteries 64, 128
ACE (see angiotensin converting enzyme)
acetylsalicylic acid 96
acute tubular necrosis (ATN) 56
age 102
aneurysm(s) 21
- abdominal aortic (AAA)
- - infrarenal 125
- - juxtarenal 125
- - pararenal 125
- aorta 55
- iliac vessels 55
- pseudoaneurysms 81
- renal artery 21, 30, 89, 90
- rupture 90, 128
angiography 2, 52, 102
- aortic 103
- intraarterial renal 22
- intravenous digital subtraction 22
- magnetic resonance 22
- renal 21, 77
- spiral computed tomographic 22
angioplasty 6, 30, 128
angiotensin I 43
angiotensin converting enzyme (ACE)
  43
- inhibitor 1, 22, 43
angiotensinogen 43
anoxic damage 43

antegrade pyelogram 107
antibiotic prophylaxis 104, 130
anticoagulant therapy 3
antihypertensive drugs 134
aortic angiography 103
aortiliac pathology 103
aorto-renal bypass surgery 83
aortography 126
arterial
- autografts 93
- flow measurements 72
artery; arteries
- accessory 64
- iliac 23
- mesenteric 51
- renal 103
- stenosis 103, 110
- suprarenal 57
- thrombosis 110
ASA (see aspirin)
aspirin (ASA) 3
asymetric stenosis 31
atherosclerosis 21
atherosclerotic disease 134
ATN (see acute tubular necrosis)
autografts, arterial 92
autonomic renal nerves, regeneration
  14, 15
autoregulation 4
autotransplant 102
autotransplantation(s) 16, 103, 111
- bilateral 102, 104
- indication 111
- renal 8, 111
autotx
- bilateral 102
- unilateral 102

B
bacteriuria 111
balloon catheter 34
bench surgery 102, 111, 135
beta blockers 3
biexponential analysis 39
bifurcations, stenosis 31
bilateral
- autotransplantation 104
- renal neoplasms 113
biopsies, serial 114
bladder papilloma, recurring 119
blood pressure 134
- regulation 8
blood, units 108
Boari flap technique 139
Boari-Ockerblad technique 141
Bricker bladder 123
bypass(es)
- extraanatomic 81
- surgery 81
- techniques, in situ 126

C
CAD (see coronary artery disease)
calcium channel blockers 3, 72
calculi
- complex 101, 102
- multiple pyelocalyceal 102
- pyelocalyceal 102
- recurrent 109
- removal, extracorporeal 109
- renal 103
- staghorn 101, 102, 111
calculous disease, renal 111
calyces 104
captopril 43
- test 22
captopril-augmented renography 44
carcinoma(s)
- renal 119
- - asychronously bilateral 115
- urothelial 111, 117f 119
cardiovascular evaluation 129
catheters, high-pressure balloon 31
celiac artery 130

cerebrospinal fluid drainage 130
chest X-ray 51
children 102
cinefilm 22
cold
- ischemia 108
- storage 59
complex calculi 101, 102
computed tomography (CT) 104, 119, 126
contralateral nonautografted kidney 109
contrast media 6, 22
- isomolar 24
- low osmolar 24
- nephrotic effects 24
- nonionic 24
coronary
- angiography 129
- artery disease (CAD) 72, 129
- artery occlusion 5
creatinine 5, 104
CT (see computed tomography)
CT angiogram 25
cultures, urine 104, 107, 108
cystinuria 103 106, 109
cystopyelogram 118
cystopyelography, retrograde 108
cystoscope, flexible 118

D
denervation, renal 10
diethylene-triamine-penta-acetate
  (DTPA) 37
dimercapto-succinic acid (DMSA) 37
diuretics 3, 130
DMSA (see dimercapto-succinic acid)
Doppler imaging 22
double-J catheter 73
drainage
- postoperative 57
- of urine 29
DTPA (see diethylene-triamine-penta-
  acetate)
duplex ultrasonography 107
dynamic studies 38

E
effective renal plasma flow (ERPF) 38
electrocardiography 51, 129
enalapril 44
end-stage renal failure 79
endartherectomy 68, 81, 95
endothelial damage 60
epidural analgesia 130
ERPF (see effectiv renal plasma flow)
ESWL (see extracorporeal shockwave lithotripsy)
Euro-Collins 102
Euro-Collins solution 60, 104, 130
ex vivo renal artery repair 95
excretion 12
external iliac artery 131
extra-anatomic bypasses 81
extracorporeal
- backtable surgery 111
- calculi removal 109
- resection 111
- shockwave lithotripsy (ESWL) 101
extremity gangrene 128
eyelid retractor 59

F
fibromuscular
- disease 127
- dysplasia 21, 79
fibrosis, periureteral 121
fistula 110
flexible cystoscope 118
fluoroscopic examinations 104
FMD 21
follow-up, postoperative 110
functional impairment 110

G
gangrene, extremity 128
Gerota's fascia 51, 56, 57, 59, 113
glomerular sclerosis 17
gonadal vein 56, 57
graft
- function, delayed 56
- loss 122

graftectomy 110
guide
- catheter 30
- wire 30

H
hematomas 43
hemodynamic monitoring 128
hemorrhage, urinary tract 110
heparin 56, 60
- low molecular 95, 96
"hibernating" 8
high-pressure balloon catheters 31
horseshoe kidneys 52
hyperfiltration 15, 17
hypertension 17, 128
- cure 95
- de novo 30
- preexistent 30
- recurrence 32
- renovascular 21
- secondary 5
hypofiltration 4
hypothermia 59, 64
hypothermic perfusion 59

I
iatrogenic ureteral defects 140
ileum interposition procedure 141
iliac artery
- external 131
- inernal 131
- vein 68
in situ bypass techniques 126
in situ tumor excision 113
incisions
- lateral (flank) 53
- skin 54, 55
- subcostal abdominal 53
- vertical midline 53
infection(s)
- chronic 102
- postoperative 111
- preoperative 108
- recurrent 102
- urinary tract 104, 111

intermesenteric nerves 9
intraarterial renal angiography 22
intravenous
- digital subtraction angiography 22
- pyelography 107
invasive stone surgery 103
irradiation injury 140
irrigation 106, 107
ischemia
- cold 108
- warm 59
ischemic nephropathy 79

J
juxtaglomerular apparatus 43

K
kidney
- contralateral 102
-- nonautografted 109
- function, rescue 5
- medullary sponge 103, 109
- replantation 66
- single 110
- size 79
- solitary 2, 111
Kocher's maneuver 58

L
life-style changes 3
lipid-lowering drugs 3
lisinopril 44
lithotomy 109
low molecular heparin 96, 97
low molecular weight dextran solution
   104
lung resection 119
lymphocele(s) 8, 29, 43

M
magnetic resonance
- angiography 22
- imaging 124

mannitol 56, 69, 130
mean transit times 43
medullary sponge kidneys 101, 109
mesenteric artery 51
metabolic disorders 103
metastases 58, 117, 121
method of Sapirstein 41
minimally invasive procedures 102
mortality
- early 122
- postoperative 82
- surgical 97, 126
multiorgan failure 133
multiple pyelocalyceal calculi 102
multiple renal arteries 51
myocardial infarction 133

N
natriuresis 14
necrosis, ureteral 56
nephrectomy 95, 102, 108, 130
- radical 57, 113
nephrocystectomy 121
nephrolithiasis 140
nephropathy, ischemic 79
nephrostomy 104, 106
- catheter 117
- tube 107
nephroureterectomy 113
nerves, intermesenteric 9

O
obstruction of urinary flow 73
OIH (see ortho-iodo-hippurate)
one functioning kidney 100
organ preservation
- perfusates 63
- techniques 63
ortho-iodo-hippurate (OIH) 38
ostial stenosis 31
oxalosis 103, 109

P
pain, debilitating 109

Palmaz stent 31
Paquin method 95
parenchyma, renal 103
patency rate 80
patient survival 126
PCNL (see percutaneous nephrolithotomy)
pelvic
- collateral circulation 68
- renal 104
percutaneous nephrolithotomy (PCNL)
   101
percutaneous transluminal renal angiography (PTRA) 2, 21
perfusates 130
- saline solutions 126
perfusion 4
- pressure 60
perioperative antibacterial prophylaxis
   64
periureteral fibrosis 121
"pigtail" catheter 22
pleura, parietal 55
Politano-Leadbetter-method 69
postoperative
- complications 101
- drainage 57
- follow-up 108
- renal insufficiency 126, 133
poststenotic dilatation 22
previous stone surgery 102
prophylactic revascularization 128
prosthetic grafts 81
pseudoaneurysms 81
psoas hitch technique 139
PTRA (see percutaneous transluminal
   renal angiography)
pulmonary function 129
pyelocalyceal calculi 102
pyelocystostomy 106, 107, 109
pyelogram, antegrade 107
pyelography 70, 107
- intravenous 107
pyeloureteric
- obstruction 110
- structure 110
pyeloureteroplasty 109

R
radical nephrectomy 57, 113
radiographic contrast agent 6
radionuclide
- renal scanning 102, 107, 128
- studies 104
radiotherapy 64
RAS (see stenosis of the renal artery)
recurrent calculi 109
recurring stone formation 109
regions of interest (ROI) 39
reinnervation 14
renal
- angiography 21, 77
- artery; arteries 103
- - accesory 128
- - aneurysms 21, 30, 88, 89
- - - rupture 91
- - collateral circulation 91
- - embolization 90
- - ex vivo repair 95, 96
- - lesion 21
- - ligation 94
- - multiple 51
- - - lesions 7
- - occlusion 52, 79, 90, 128, 140
- - perfusion 126
- - reconstruction 95
- - single functioning kidney 7
- - stenosis 7, 21, 31
- - surgery 123
- - thrombosis 28, 91
- autotransplantation 111
- calculi 103
- calculous disease 111
- carcinoma 119
- - asychronously bilateral 115
- clamp time 126
- denervation 10
- dysfunction 78
- failure 17, 21
- - end-stage 79
- flow 102
- function 102
- - conversation 123
- - impaired 120
- - threatened 101

renal
- functional reserve 16
- ischemia 125
- nonfunction 102
- parenchyma 103
- parenchymal pathology 104
- pelvis 104
- scintigraphy 78
- vasculature 51
- vasoconstriction 10
- vein 68
- - thrombosis 120, 140
renin 1, 10, 43, 78
- determination 22
renography 1, 37
- captopril-augmented 43
renoprotective effects 17
renovascular hypertension (RVH) 1, 21, 78
reoperation 110
resection area 114
resistive index 26
respiratory disease 51
retention 12
retractor
- eyelid 59
- self-retaining 55
retrograde cystopyelography 108
retroperitoneal fibrosis 64, 139, 140
revascularization 2, 6, 23, 104
Ringer's acetate 72, 130
Ringer's lactate 60
ROI (see regions of interest)
RVH (see renovascular hypertension)

S
salt 8, 12
- depletion 13
- excretion 12
saphenous vein 93
Schlegel method 40
scintigraphy, renal 78
secondary hypertension 5
segmental arteries stenosis 31
sepsis 133
septicemia 120, 140

serum creatinine 79, 102
single compartment model 39
single kidney 110
skin incision 54, 55
solitary kidney 2, 111
spinal cord damage 130
spiral computed tomographic angiography 22
split renal functions 41, 95
staghorn calculi 101, 102, 111
stenosis
- artery 110
- asymetric 31
- bifurcations 31
- ostial 31
- renal artery (RAS) 31, 77
- - prevalence 77
- segmental arteries 31
stent 3
stone(s)
- formation 111
- - reccuring 109
- producers, chronic 111
- recurrence 101, 111
- removal 101
- residual 101
- surgery, invasive 103
structure, pyeloureteric 110
superior mesenteric artery 130
suprarenal
- aortic clamping 125
- artery 57
- vein 56
surgery 6
surgical mortality 126
sympathetic innervation 9

T
Takayasu's arteritis 21
technetium-99m generator 37
thallium scanning 129
thrombectomy 120
thrombosis
- artery 110
- prophylaxis 96
- renal

- - artery 28
- - vein 28, 120, 140
total effective renal plasma flow (ERPF) 104
transstenotic pressure gradient 22, 30
transureteroureteric 139
transurethral resection 119
tube, nephrostomy 107
tuberculosis 102
tubular 15
- necrosis 120
- - acute (ATN) 56
tumor
- bed 114
- excision, in situ 113
- free margins 112
- reccurence 119, 121

U
ultrasonography 104, 132
- duplex 107
ureter 104
- arterial supply 53
- blood supply 65
- intramural part 122
- necrosis 65
- stricture 140
ureteral
- defects, iatrogenic 140
- injury 139
- necrosis 56
- obstruction 132
ureterocystostomy, re-doing 73
ureterolysis 121
ureteroneocystostomy 104, 131
ureteroscopy (URS) 101, 123
urinary
- calculous disease 111
- flow 95
- infections, therapy-resistant 141
- leaks 43

- tract
- - hemorrhage 110
- - infection 104, 111
- - - chronic 108
- - - recurrent 108
- reconstruction 69
urine
- cultures 104, 107, 108
- drainage 29
- flow 29
- leakage 29
urinomas 43
urography 104, 132
urothelial carcinoma 113, 117*f* 119
URS (see ureteroscopy)

V
vascular
- obstruction 43
- spasm 56
vasculature, renal 51
vasoconstriction, renal 10
vasospasm 72
vein(s)
- external internal iliac 68
- gonadal 56, 57
- multiple 52
- renal 68
- saphenous 92
- suprarenal 56
- thrombosis 28
vena cava 51
venography 67
visceral vessels 125

W
warm ischemia 59
water 12
- excretion 12

Printing: Saladruck, Berlin
Binding: Buchbinderei Lüderitz & Bauer, Berlin